Nature's Pathways to Womb-Wellness
A Journey Towards Fibroid Elimination

Imani Sorhaindo
(Auraum Benneurt)

Ba Hons, PGCE and Diploma in Holistic Health

Copyright © 2021 Imani Sorhaindo, KMT Rising Ltd. All rights reserved.

No part of this publication may be reproduced, stored in a retrieval system or transmitted in any form or by any means, electronic, mechanical, photocopying, recording, storage or otherwise, without the prior permission of the author.

Front and back cover design by Kitwana of Nefer Graphics.
nefergraphics@gmail.com

Breathe...
And you will know just how to heal yourself.
In the soft, quietude of the mind,
Silken your breath.
Here, you will learn to glide across the satin sheets
Of life!
Breathe...
And you will re-member this blueprint;
The keys to unlock each bolted door;
The salve for your damaged wounds.
Search for it!
Breathe...

By Imani Sorhaindo (Auraum Benneurt)

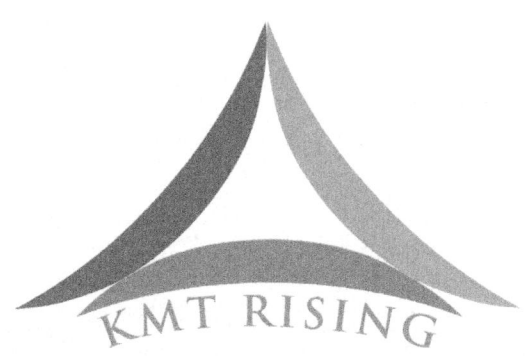

∞
FOREWORD

There has been a history of struggles for black women across the globe battling fibroids for a number of decades. The quest to learn, heal and survive the detrimental impact of the condition, has made way for practitioners to come forth to support sisters on their journey to better health. In this seminal work, Imani Sorhaindo presents her research, the lived experiences of women she has worked with and her own personal journey of living with fibroids.

Women's health advocates across the globe have highlighted the need for more attention to be given to this condition that causes much heart ache for women and in some cases their families, loved ones and employers too. To borrow from an old Congolese proverb, 'a single bracelet does not jingle'. Fibroids brought healthcare practitioners and advocates together from UK, Caribbean, Africa, Europe and USA to form the Global Fibroid Alliance in 2019. It is here where I continue to work with Imani and others as dedicated members who wish to see political change for women living with fibroids.

In 2016, my organisation Noire Wellness began to focus on fibroids and it is here where I learned of the some 80% of women that have fibroids, through the work of our partners at Lake Health and Wellbeing. I was humbled to have met sister Imani before then, at the community Taui Network gatherings, where we would learn about our true systems of spirituality and later had the pleasure of experiencing her delivery of work on our *Fibroid Series Programme*.

It is against this background that sister Imani has carefully created her long awaited book of hugely valuable insight into fibroids. She does so fully aware that there are many women that continue to battle the condition. The public health and wider studies into fibroids have long been documented, however none have tackled the issue in such a delicate, spirited and hopeful way as sister Imani does here.

Sister Imani reminds us that while sharing the highs and lows of her own journey, that no experience will be the same and that women must seek support and guidance from within the love and richness of the communities and families that surround them. In the past, and even now still, women of the motherland have traditionally used mother earth to heal most ailments and so after decades of growing up in the western world, in chapter 7, sister Imani reminds us of the need and space for a holistic approach to eliminating fibroids.

We have lost so many of our ancient traditions, and reclaiming some of these forms the foundation of sister Imani Sorhaindo's book, *Nature's Pathways to Womb-Wellness*. She reminds us that we have the truth in our hands if only we embrace the teachings, lessons and shared experiences of highly skilled and knowledgeable practitioners such as her. Sister Imani Sorhaindo has written with clarity and her work is an inspiration to readers who seek more depth on their journey of fibroid elimination. It is one that I am proud to support and truly believe that we must all share her insights within our communities to help heal our mothers, daughters, sisters, nieces and aunties. The journey must go on.

Candice Bryan, BA (hons), MSc and founder of Noire Wellness based in London UK

ACKNOWLEDGEMENTS

I thank Neter (God) for life and the talents gifted to me and I hope this body of research, coupled with my own journey of healing through fibroids, along with the experiences of hundreds of women I have worked to support, will contribute to women's wellness and healing across the globe. Only when women are better-informed about their health and are placed central in their own health care plans, will we experience a paradigm shift in achieving vitality and longevity. With a blueprint to guide us to mindful living we can then begin to address the planet's earth-shattering cries for peace, harmony, and ultimate healing.

I am humbly indebted to Shekhem Ur Shekhem Ra Un Nefer Amen, the Great Sage, High priest and author of the *Metu Neter Volumes 1 to 7*, *Maat 11 Laws*, *Healing is in the Spirit* and many other books, who has restored the ancient Egyptian (Ausarian) teachings. These fundamentals centred around the universal laws governing all life activity, coupled with life-force energy (qi) cultivation, have allowed me access to a blueprint which has enabled me to direct my life positively and holistically towards all-round success. Tua U (Thank you).

I also want to say Tua U to Ur Aua Khem Men Sih Napata, beloved King, Counsellor, Healer and health practitioner and dear friend, who has shown me a living example of what sacrifice and devotion really looks like. As I meditate, improve my health, respond to life challenges from a place of peace, as I strive to work daily to cultivate my life-force, I marvel on all I have learnt through your instruction and living example. I am indebted to you for your leadership, guidance, love, patience, and tenacity, in wanting to ensure that people of the world return to truth and an elevated way of living. Thank you for your holistic, intuitive health counsel over the years.

Thank you to you, the readers of this book, for calling this book into your life. It is a book birthed out of my primal urge to nurture and heal myself and others, living in the knowledge that returning to a more natural and holistic way of life contributes to wellness significantly.

To my family and friends, thank you for your love, encouragement, and patience as I sacrificed time away from many of you, so that I can write. Thank you for your tremendous trust and confidence in me throughout my life journey as a daughter, sister, mother, aunt, grandmother, relative, priestess, community leader, friend, colleague, and teacher. I hope you have benefited in some meaningful way by eating some of the fruits of the tree which has nourished me emotionally, culturally, and spiritually over the years. Our phone calls and face-to-face conversations about life, health, love, spirituality and addressing health inequalities have surely strengthened me, and I hope they have strengthened you too.

Last, but certainly not least, to everyone who has contributed their amazing life stories to the shaping of this book; the women who lived or are living with fibroids daily and just keep going despite the high levels of discomfort and pain; the many women who completed questionnaires to inform the research necessary for the book; the women who participated and shared their stories during the fibroid support groups where we all learnt to become more honest, trusting and 'real' with each other as sisters; and for those who attended my lectures, events, and Twitter chat interviews, around the topics of Fibroids and Womb-Wellness; Thank you!

Thank you to the doctors and other health practitioners who were receptive to being interviewed. Many of you saw health inequalities in your workplace and felt moved to speak out. Thank you for all these courageous acts!

Although this book is primarily for women, I fully appreciate the millions of men who have contributed and continue to contribute to women's health improvements and support women during their fibroid journeys. Whether you are the husbands, fathers, uncles, brothers, nephews, sons, friends, or health practitioners in our lives, I want to say thank you. I urge you to continue to appreciate us and value the essential role we too play in society. We walk beside you as essential parts of a whole.

Hetep (Peace)

Auraum Benneurt (Imani Sorhaindo) - 24th August 2017

INTRODUCTION

I first found out I had fibroids around 2005, when I was 37 years old. I was creaming my body and noticed a small lump below the surface of my womb area. I grew anxious and booked an urgent appointment with my doctor, only to be told that I probably had fibroids. A few weeks later I was invited to have a scan, which displayed three fibroids, 3-5cm in size. In the consultation room I started pouring out all my health complaints which I had bottled up for a few years, thinking they were just normal trials women had to endure. I spoke of the pain and discomfort during menses, the heavy bleeding and heavy clotting, but I soon realised that the consultant was not actively listening and not responding to my need to share the details of what I was going through. All those years I had been unaware that so many of the physical problems and discomforts I had been experiencing, that had left me feeling exhausted trying to juggle family life, voluntary work, and a full-time managerial job, all that physical and emotional havoc in my life, were caused by these entities, just 3cms or so in size.

The consultant just stared at me, did not ask me any probing questions about my symptoms and then stated that in his opinion, the best thing for me at my age was a hysterectomy. I was shocked by his response, intuitively sensing there must be another way. I composed myself and had to 'ban my belly' as they say in Jamaica, brace myself not to react, and try and listen to his advice. I asked myself, was this the default rhetoric offered to women when they came to his surgery with fibroids? During those moments, I felt unsupported and unheard. At that point, to me, it became so much more than about the fibroids themselves, but about my life choices. I was treated as though the fibroids were 'things' that just had to be rooted out and my problems would go away. I was offered no explanation as to the cause; I needed to know how they came into being. There was a lack of understanding that there must be a deeper reason for their growth in the first place.

I continued to have this internal chat with myself as the consultant started to write down his notes, looking up at his computer screen periodically. I could feel my hands and stomach getting hot and I felt a twisting sensation in my lower abdomen due to my level of discomfort. I then blurted out, "I don't want a hysterectomy!" He looked at me perplexed and continued asserting his view that it was the best treatment in my situation, me being "a grandmother after all". This just added insult to injury, and I recall my last words to him, "…doctor, let us direct the focus of this discussion to *my healing and not on a hysterectomy. I don't want that!*"

Nine months later, having pressed on to try and get a second opinion, I returned to see another consultant, only to now find that there were another three fibroids taking up residence in my sacred womb, declaring squatters' rights. I felt alone and without answers, but at least this time there were some alternative treatments offered to me such as a myomectomy or embolisation. I was clear that I did not want to have a hysterectomy, I wanted to keep open the possibility of conceiving a child should I choose to, but when I asked whether there were any other options such as more natural and less invasive treatments, there were no answers.

Walking home after this second appointment, it was then it finally sunk in, and it dawned on me that I was looking for answers in the wrong place, and with the wrong practitioners. The GPs and consultants were doing their job and that was to treat this condition. They could not assist me to explore the causative factors of how the fibroids were created, nor direct me to holistic pathways to eliminate them; in fact, many seemed antagonistic to complementary or alternative approaches and so were not receptive when I made an appeal for this consideration.

It was in those quiet moments that something started to take root inside me, an idea whose time had come. I started to feel a strong stirring of determination as I grew to realise that healing my fibroids starts with me. It was my responsibility to search for these answers on how to eliminate fibroids, it was my responsibility to start listening to my inner guide as to what needed to change in my life, to get answers on how to heal myself, and to do so naturally.

During this time, I was reading a best-selling book called *Metu Neter Volume 1*, by Ra Un Nefer Amen. In it, he wrote a statement that ignited my interest in health and longevity and allowed me to start appreciating the interrelationship between peace, oneness, health, and success. He spoke about there being 11 fundamental laws which governed life itself. He wrote, "We live in a world that was created, and is maintained by a *unified* working of a *multiplicity* of agencies. We live in a world that is composed of a multiplicity of entities that are unified through a web of interdependence." I sat and marvelled at the profoundness of this statement, contemplating on the reality that everything on this planet is involved in an inter-connected dance, and therefore is pulled towards bringing itself back to its original source, peace. For me, this meant that in the context of my health improvements, finding this equilibrium in my life was going to be critical. My life was certainly not balanced, and this realisation was the moment of change for me.

When our life displays imbalance, and mind, body and spirit are not cooperating as a balanced whole, it is because in one way or another we have abdicated our responsibility and duty of care to ourselves, which often includes leaving our healthcare fully in the hands of others. This is evident in the life choices we make; what we put in and onto our bodies, what we feed our minds, the way we eat, when we eat, how we breathe and the daily activities we are engrossed in. As a result of prolonged unhealthy choices, an array of problems emerge which start to attack our internal body-system. Where else can our health go but downhill from there, spiralling down the road of stagnation, decay, and eventual disease!

To compound the fibroids situation, there is a lack of robust mainstream research available to guide women through this maze. We often struggle to locate scientific research that outlines the multiple causes of feminine un-wellness, and struggle even more to get mainstream access to holistic therapies and treatments to help us address our symptoms, whilst preserving our wombs. Yes, let us tell it as it is, we live in a world that by and large, does not promote complementary and holistic approaches, and we are paying the price. We are in an age of such technical advancement, and yet we see higher numbers in our communities with diabetes, bowel and prostate cancer, fibroids, lupus, high blood pressure and a list of other non-communicable diseases (NCD's). Why should this be?

In today's so-called modern world here in the UK, we are presented with a bountiful, diverse platter which encourages gluttony, and I do not just mean food. Regardless of who we are, we are encouraged to over-shop, overeat, and over emote. We eat what we want, when we want, how we want it, without a holistic and healthy framework to guide us. We interact with millions of toxins each day and spout assertively, that we have 'free-choice'. We need to ask the questions, are we really using free choice or are we acting on compulsion and addiction? Have we become slaves to our taste buds which cannot discern what is good or bad for us? We inflict ourselves, and our families, with high levels of salt and sugar, and our sensual cravings drive us to make so many unhealthy choices as we yearn for that next 'high', often trying to satisfy an underlying sense of unfulfillment.

These external and internal voices telling us to eat more, accumulate more, buy more, look this way, want more, and yet for many women I work with, there is still a feeling of discontent. Let us stop and ask ourselves, where is this sense of dissatisfaction coming from? Fibroids cannot be cured without us first examining our ideas about our self-image, our health, vitality, and lifestyle choices, and addressing the level of disconnection between the above aspects of our lives.

A linear way of looking at resolving fibroids means trying to cut out the fibroids as opposed to looking at the root cause, and so, in many cases the fibroids will grow back and they will continue to have deleterious consequences for women's health and well-being, and consequently the health and well-being of our nations. This is the reason why a call for a holistic view of health and healing is needed at this time.

In 2012 to 2013, in England alone, health service documentation outlined that there were over 30,000 hysterectomies carried out due to the formation and acceleration of uterine fibroid masses. In the United States, hysterectomy is the second most frequently performed surgical procedure for all women of reproductive age, with approximately 600,000 hysterectomies carried out annually. The leading cause of hysterectomy is leiomyomas (fibroids) followed by endometriosis and uterine prolapse. (Keshavarz et al., 2002; Wilcox et al., 1994).

In 2015, the Unison National Women's Conference in UK, highlighted that "Black women suffer disproportionately from fibroids and are three to five times more likely to develop them than white women". The Unison report also highlighted that fibroids are the main reason behind 30% of hysterectomies in white women and over 50% of hysterectomies in Black women.

This whole issue made me stop in my tracks and consider the number of women across the globe being denied the right to a high quality of life, and in many cases, the right to retain their womb. It spurred me on to do this work to assist in the healing of women. Whilst undertaking research for this book, I formally interviewed 25 women of African and Caribbean origin, and had also spoken to many women over the years about fibroids and womb-wellness, and the health disparities were glaring. It propelled me to investigate further what was impacting the lives of so many women to lead to fibroids; why were there such high incidents of fibroids and were there any examples of medical apartheid affecting women disproportionality, preventing such a high number of Black women from bringing back future generations to come. I know it sounds rather deep and you may wish to pause for a moment to allow this all to sink in, but I ask that we all ask lots of questions as we start to embark on this journey to heal ourselves.

For me, the journey started when I began to appreciate that disease does not take place in a vacuum. We are active participants in determining our health, wellness, and vitality, but we are not taught some essential aspects about life and living. Factors such as lifestyle, diet, nutrition, exercise, thoughts, negative emotions, in addition to our physical environment and genetic history, all play a part in determining the level of life-force energy (qi) we have available in order for us to heal, reap, harvest, and actualise our dreams and goals.

I suspected that there were many other women suffering in silence with this condition around the world, and so I felt called to set up a fibroid support group. Slowly at first, but soon drastically increasing, Black sisters started making contact and started attending. The work to reach and support women led to my gaining a Diploma in Holistic Healthcare, and then more recently a Diploma in Acupressure. It also led to me being invited to lecture and speak on the topic of fibroids at national and international platforms, becoming one of the founder members of the Global Fibroids Alliance to set up campaigns to get the message out there that women wanted answers, women wanted healing. In 2019, I was elated to give my first fibroid lecture in Dominica, West Indies, where I was born. From such a desperate and challenging personal situation, fibroid elimination became a life mission, and it has been a blessing to assist so many women to work towards healing themselves.

I would ask anyone reading this book to first start by allowing your life to be one which seeks to transcend fear, anger, jealousy, envy, disunity, and dis-ease. There are many of us who are crippled by these emotions, as well as by self-hate and self-neglect. All these lead to imbalances in our being and eventually disease. We can transcend these negative emotions by focusing less on the materialistic and trivial aspects of life and by starting the inner journey towards mindful, purposeful, and authentic living. This will allow us all to make healthier choices about what thoughts we accept and dwell on, what food we eat, what water we drink, what exercise we do, how and when we interact with nature, with ourselves and others, and what type of relationships we draw near to us; knowing that holistic wealth, health, and success are biproducts of our oneness with all. I believe success and optimum health in life are assured when we live our essential nature, which is peace. But how do we get there? We can start this journey a step at a time by educating ourselves about how to create a lifestyle that is not diametrically opposed to nature, and the best time to start is now!

DISCLAIMER

The strategies, techniques and considerations outlined in this book are for informational purposes only. The author is not rendering medical advice, diagnosis, nor are they prescribing or treating any disease or condition. The book is an aid towards enabling the reader to make more informed choices in relation to their general health, well-being, and pathways to longevity, more specifically, towards womb-wellness. It is imperative that before beginning any revised health, nutrition or exercise programme, the reader receives full medical clearance from their doctor or health practitioner.

CONTENTS

	Foreword	iv
	Acknowledgements	vi
	Introduction	viii
Chapter 1	What Are Fibroids?	1

- Fibroid Sizes and Types

Chapter 2	Symptoms and Detection	4
Chapter 3	The Risks and Causative Factors	9

- Toxins – The Pathway to Dis-ease
- Oestrogen Dominance, the Endocrine System, and the Adrenals
- Obesity, Weight Management and Fibroids
- Acidic Food
- I need my SUGAR!
- Genetically Modified Organisms (GMOs)
- Growth Hormones in Meat and Dairy Products
- To Soy or Not to Soy
- Environmental and Household Toxins
- Our Emotions – "I'm only human after all!"
- The Stress Response
- Suppression and Pushing Down Trauma

Chapter 4	Black Women and Fibroids	33

- Ideological and Systemic Racism
- Combat Fatigue – "I am tired of playing Cultural Expert"
- Black Hair Relaxers

Chapter 5	My Work with Black Women with Fibroids	42

| Chapter 6 | Conventional Treatments for Fibroids | 47 |

- Hysterectomy
- Myomectomy
- Uterine Artery Embolization (UAE)
- Magnetic Resonance Imaging (MRI) and Other Treatments
- Drug Treatments

| Chapter 7 | Holistic Approaches to Fibroid Elimination | 52 |

- Creating a Feminine Internal Environment
- Traditional Chinese Medicine (TCM)
- Energy Balancing and Its Health Benefits
- Love and the Energetic Impact of Emotions on Health
- Hydration – Water, Water Everywhere
- Meditation and Breathwork
- Cultivating Mindfulness in Meditation
- The Deep Sleep
- A Relationship with Self – Tuning in and Body Awareness
- Feminine Sexual Energy
- Inducing Joy

| Chapter 8 | Diet, Nutrition and Supplementation | 71 |

- We Become What We Eat
- Mindful Eating
- Nutritional Therapy
- Supplementation

| Chapter 9 | Concluding Remarks - A Wake-Up Call for Health and Wellness | 80 |

- Getting Started – A Checklist for Fibroid Elimination

Appendix 1 Useful Resources	85
Appendix 2 Bibliography	88
Index	93

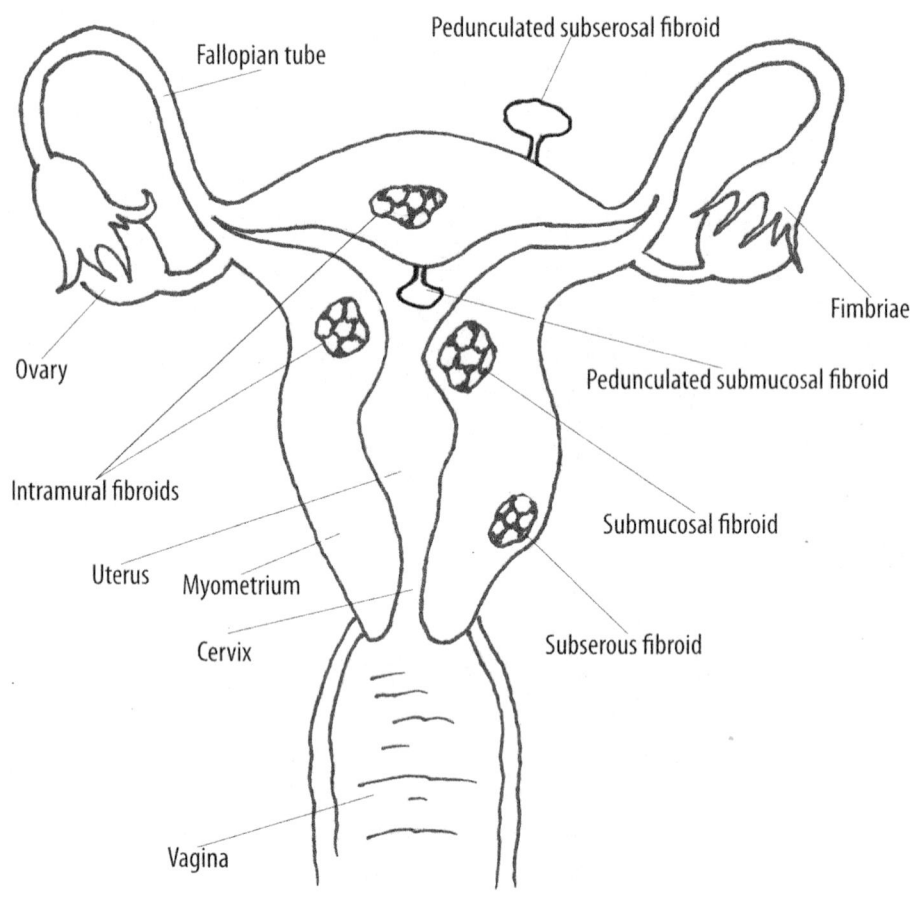

Fibroids illustration by Carol Sorhaindo

CHAPTER 1
What Are Fibroids?

Let us start from the beginning and introduce ourselves to these masses called FIBROIDS. If you have them, please try not to harbour any negative emotions about having them, as this will just make matters worse. Instead, stay peaceful and start that journey towards healing and self-empowerment. They certainly will not go away on their own, nor will they go away by directing negative energy towards them and cursing their existence like many women have done before. That amount of stress and negative energetic vibration will further contribute to their growth. The initial step to transforming our lives to wellness is first of all, accepting that something needs to change, then we can start on the journey towards self-love; understanding how the mind, body and spirit is pro-success when we align ourselves with that synchronicity.

Fibroids are the most common, non-cancerous, mass in a woman's reproductive system and are composed of the same smooth muscle tissue as the womb. They are also referred to as leiomyomatas, leiomyomas, fibromyomas or myomas. Many Traditional Chinese Medicine (TCM) specialists see this 'rogue' tissue as nature's clever way of isolating and protecting the main organs in the body system from any toxins, which cannot be disposed of through the usual elimination processes, due to health imbalances.

1 in 5 women will develop fibroids at some point in their life and this is a growing concern. During the perimenopausal stage (between 41-45 years) fibroids tend to increase significantly in size and will then tend to shrink during the menopausal stage because of a decrease in oestrogen.

In most cases fibroids locate themselves in the smooth muscle fibre of the myometrium in the uterus and in their early stages of development, they can appear soft and movable. As they grow, they can become very dense and hard, like stone. When we look to conventional medicine, there is little shared about the causes of fibroids, and so the treatments offered tend to steer towards invasive surgery or shrinking them with pharmaceutical drugs. TCM however, has a more extensive body of research around the causes of such masses, and considers more holistic approaches to eliminate them.

The size of a fibroid mass can range from pea-size to watermelon-size, and they can grow singly or in grape-like clusters, within or on the outside of the uterus. They can start to grow in women as young as 19, but in most cases, they tend to grow when women are in their mid-30s to mid-40s.

Fibroid Sizes

The sizes of fibroids in comparison to foetus sizes, gestation weeks and various fruit (approximations).

3.0 inch	Standard size of the uterus	Small pear or apple
3.5 inch	10-week pregnancy size	Orange
4.5 inch	12-week pregnancy size	Grapefruit
6.3 inch	16-week pregnancy size	Melon
8.7 inch	22-week pregnancy size	Pineapple
10.5 inch	28-week pregnancy size	Pumpkin

Fibroid Types

There are four types of fibroids, and some women have the full range of all four types in and around the uterus. If you do have fibroids, it is important to get to know which type/s you have, as the suggested treatment options may vary based on type and location.

Intramural fibroids are located entirely within the muscle layer of the uterine wall. These grow in the wall of the womb and records show that this tends to be the most frequently identified fibroid. Intramural masses can distort and enlarge the internal cavity of the womb; giving the area a globular feeling which makes women look like they are in the early stages of pregnancy.

Subserosal or **Subserous** fibroids develop and project themselves from the outer surface of the womb. They grow on the outer layer of the womb wall and can often grow on stalks. These fibroids are also termed pedunculated fibroids. They can grow to a large size, but usually do not directly affect the size of the womb and its capacity. More likely, they start to place pressure on the bladder and rectal area making it uncomfortable for many women.

One of the least common are **Submucosal** or **Submucous** fibroids, which make up about 5% of the fibroids researched. They develop in the muscle underneath the inner lining of the womb and grow into the womb cavity. These fibroids can greatly disrupt the shape of the womb and can lead to diarrhoea, excessive bleeding, incontinence, or actual kidney impairments. Oftentimes these masses can also grow on pedunculated stalks inside the womb, and if long enough, they can hang down into the cervix area or can even start growing out of the cervix, causing all types of fertility problems.

Finally, there are the **Cervical** fibroids which are also quite rare, and they tend to grow in the neck of the womb. A few of the clients I have supported have complained of painful intercourse with this type of fibroid. These are often difficult to remove with surgery without damaging the surrounding area.

CHAPTER 2
Symptoms and Detection

Approximately 25-50% of women with fibroids are symptomatic, experiencing mild to severe symptoms, some of which are listed above under fibroid types. Symptoms may also include heavy, painful and/or prolonged menses, bleeding in between menses, passing of clots, severe mood swings, increased urinary frequency, pelvic pain, lower back pain, intense pressure on the bladder or rectal area, abdominal pain, cramps, and anaemia. Personally, I also experienced an adult type of acne due to hormonal imbalance, physical exhaustion, and nervous system imbalance which led to irritability and impatience, during the early stages of my fibroid growth. Some women also found that their fibroids greatly impacted on their levels of intimacy, due to discomfort whilst having sex.

One of problems with fibroids is that they are inherently difficult to detect physically by touch, and by the time you can actually feel them, they may have already become hardened, making them more difficult to eliminate. Also, there are not a specific set of common symptoms that 100% indicate fibroids as the likely cause. Fibroids impact women in different ways. It is therefore important to closely monitor any changes in your emotional and mental health, or any physical changes, and report those of concern to your GP or health practitioner as early as possible; or adopt a lifestyle that mitigates the risk of fibroids forming in the first place.

Growing up in the Caribbean, creaming my body was a regular daily ritual and one I continued in England as the weather dried out my skin. As mentioned in my introduction, it was during this daily ritual that I first detected my fibroids. This is one method of self-detection of fibroids, regularly massaging or gently stroking your stomach area and checking for new lumps and bumps or changes to existing ones. Although by this stage the fibroid may have grown large and calcified so it is better to speak to your GP as soon as possible.

If fibroids are suspected, your GP would normally suggest an ultrasound scan to accurately confirm and diagnose fibroids. Make sure you bring a notepad and pen and ask lots of questions about the size, location and type of fibroid because all of this is important in the treatment of your fibroids.

Fibroids may also be associated with reproductive problems, infertility, and challenges during pregnancy, which could include miscarriage or preterm pregnancy. Some women have also shared how they started to develop a negative body-image as the fibroids grew larger, and clothes no longer fitted. It was not uncommon for women to be asked by family and friends whether they were pregnant, because of their protruding tummy. So, we can see from some of the symptoms above, that fibroids are known to severely disrupt the quality of life, confidence, and vitality of many women.

If left untreated, fibroids can grow so large that they outgrow their own blood supply, resulting in anaemia or a process of degeneration termed *hyaline degeneration*. This degeneration can encourage an over-production of calcium, whereby the fibroid hardens. The formation of this hardened calcium shell around the fibroid mass can cause a great deal of pain, discomfort, and pressure. It is during this calcification stage, that the fibroid tends to be most prominent, making it easier to detect upon examination. This is often the stage where, due to calcification, it can become more difficult to eliminate fibroids using natural treatments, but not impossible.

98% of the women I have worked with who had fibroids, were not aware that they needed to rejuvenate their blood after each cycle of their menses, due to the significant amount of blood loss during this time. Energy and vital nutrients are lost, and additional herbs and supplementation are required to help restore the quality and efficient supply of life-giving blood. It is the vitality of our blood which also determines the quality of energy we store in our body, to carry out our day-to-day functions; so, you can imagine the impact this has on so many women who are dealing with heavy menstrual cycles at home or in their places of employment. Many women experience anaemia or light-headedness, as the fibroids often tend to divert an amount of oxygenated blood that would usually go to the uterus area, to other parts of the body.

We can therefore see why there can be no 'one-size fits all' approach to treating fibroids, and why we need to fully understand which fibroids are in our body when visiting the gynaecologist, to aid us with our decision making about what treatment, if any, to undertake. We also need to gain more understanding as to the range of causal factors which lead to fibroid growth before deciding to cut them out. The fibroid is the symptom and not the cause, so they are more than likely to grow back if we do not get to the root of the health problem.

During a population-based observational study of 737,638 women aged 15-54 by The Health Improvement Network (THIN) in 2000-2009, it was concluded that women with fibroids, or symptoms suggestive of fibroids, experience significant distress that reduces their quality of life, particularly women of minority ethnic communities and women in the lower income bracket. The findings also concluded that many women were likely undiagnosed, highlighting the need for improved awareness and education in the community around this subject. Fibroids were confirmed in a high proportion of the women who had the code UF (Uterine Fibroid) upon diagnosis, however a significant further two-thirds of fibroid cases were identified in women who were only coded as 'hysterectomies', despite their fibroids being the main reason for the invasive hysterectomy. This highlights that fibroids are going under-reported due to mis-coding or incorrect coding by many primary care physicians. It also draws attention to many physicians coding the *symptoms* of fibroids and not fibroids itself, which makes it difficult to obtain accurate data. This seems to be the case both in the UK and the US, and based on this research I am concerned that fibroid cases are significantly higher than currently being reported.

The 'watch and wait' approach has not proved to be the best form of guidance to women upon their first detection of fibroids. The view is often taken that if the patient is not experiencing severe pain, discomfort, or complications, then the fibroids can just be left alone. Reassuring statements such as, "don't worry, we will just keep an eye on it" or "you don't need to worry because it's quite small", were common phrases shared by women who I have supported over the years, however, when fibroids were left untreated, for the vast majority, they grew significantly and were then more difficult to eliminate.

It is estimated that around 20-30% of the world's population of women have or have had fibroids, but recent studies show that this is a very conservative figure. In reality, we may be looking at figures of 50-60% if we consider that many women may not even be aware that they have fibroids, due to the size of the fibroid or due to not experiencing any severe symptoms.

The *Fibroid Growth Study* in the US highlighted in 2013 that there was more than $4,600 spent in health care costs during the first year of a woman's diagnosis of their fibroids. This would include consultations and ultrasounds scans. This study also went on to add that the national medical costs associated with fibroids exceeds $2 billion annually and that women of African origin have a significantly higher fibroid incidence rate than white women, with a threefold higher risk of hysterectomies. We are also now seeing significant growth and acceleration rates of fibroids in the UK, the Caribbean islands and in the continent of Africa.

In 2010, comparisons were made across the globe in relation to fibroid cases, with China and Japan having the lowest rates. These lower rates were attributed to the good sources of soy in their diet, coming from fermented foods such as miso, natto, tofu, dried soybeans, and the high levels of iodine in their diet, from sea vegetables and seaweeds such as Nori. In 2015, another study showed a significant rise in fibroid growth in China and Japan, and this was attributed to an insurgence of western diet and processed foods into the Asian market. It is not surprising that scientists are now observing accelerated patterns of disease generally mirroring that of the US and UK; with a significant variance between city dwellers and non-city dwellers; often showing a 40-50% increase of fibroids amongst city-dwellers. This is likely due to the same challenges we face across the globe now, with an increase in environmental toxins and fast foods.

At this time, I would ask you to pause for thought as you read these statistics and get a sense of the cumulative and rippling effects, when 50-60% of the female population is experiencing this level of womb un-wellness and still having to just 'get on with life'. What does this mean in terms of our ability to generate the energy to consistently manage and support ourselves, our families, and our communities; what is the impact on our nations, on the world? What is the price paid overall when we do not pay attention to our health and well-being?

The statistics from an American community survey cited in the *Journal of Women's Health, Vol. 27, No. 11, November 2018*, stated there were approximately 11 million women diagnosed with fibroids in the US alone, 30% underwent surgical hysterectomy, myomectomy, or endometrial ablation, or procedural treatment, and 71% used pharmacologic treatments (over the counter pain relief, iron supplements, hormonal contraceptives), to help alleviate symptoms. One survey documented that it took women 3-4 years to seek treatment, and about 50% of women saw at least two healthcare providers before they were diagnosed with fibroids. The survey also highlighted that Black women were more interested in uterine-preserving options. Preserving the ability to have children, relieving symptoms such as heavy bleeding, and regaining energy, represented the significant unmet needs for suitable treatments. In the UK there is a significant lack of data which breaks down ethnicity, for there to be robust comparisons made. As previously indicated, this may be due to under-recording and/or incorrect recording, amongst primary care physicians in the UK, as they tend to record the reason as the symptoms of uterine fibroids, more often than recording and coding an actual diagnosis of UF.

Fibroids are serious in terms of our overall health, quality of life, vitality, and reproductive health. The facts that cannot be ignored are:

1. We need to acknowledge that there are many causative factors which impact on their formation and acceleration,

2. 1 in 5 women (statistics increase to 1 in 3 for Black women) have experienced fibroids at some point in their life; so, it is progressive enough to warrant more extensive research and analysis,

3. Women need to be better educated about the variety of effective holistic and complementary treatments available and not just the conventional ones, in order to make informed choices,

4. Fibroids can be reduced and eliminated through a range of holistic and non-invasive intervention.

There is certainly a need for early investigation and intervention regarding fibroids, as in my years of supporting women, the majority have been referred to me quite late in the fibroid growth stage, resulting in increased health complications, pain, and discomfort, due to their fibroids being left untreated for years.

It is encouraging to know that there are many holistic approaches and treatments available to women, as well as the more conventional treatments, and one of my aims is to ensure more women have access to more information, in order to make informed choices. It is also important for women to spend more time doing their own research, speaking to holistic health practitioners as well as conventional doctors, as part of their journey towards womb-wellness.

CHAPTER 3
The Risks and Causative Factors

Toxins – The Pathway to Dis-ease

When we think of the word *toxins* we often only think about external, environmental chemicals alone, and can feel a sense of powerlessness when trying to address this global issue. However, there are a host of other toxins flooding our system daily which we have more power and influence over, but first we need to understand what is meant by the word *toxin* itself.

Toxins mainly refer to any compound which can have a negative impact on our cells and cellular structure. These can be exotoxins or endotoxins. Exotoxins refer to externally derived pollutants, synthetic chemicals and heavy metals which have a negative impact on our health. However, there are endotoxins which are produced by the body, such as the end products of metabolism, free radicals which are generated during the detoxification process, or by-products released from the intestinal tract bacteria. These also need effective elimination from our body system. If our liver is impaired or our gut is not healthy, this will reduce our body's ability to heal, if left unaddressed.

We are one inter-connected web, and so as we continue to pollute the earth, in turn, we pollute our body system. The planet has become saturated with the residues of harmful chemicals, due to our demands for all the things that we want and need, and as a result, toxicity has become a primary driver to disease. Toxins can seep into our life support systems, i.e. the soil, the air, foods, the water, into our body system, including our mind.

We are bombarded with so many different types of foods, packaged in so many different and alluring ways, that it is often difficult to know what is nutritious and healthy for us, and what is not. We are told one thing after the other, and if truth be told, we are confused! We also need to be mindful of the wide range of harmful foods creeping into the organic and vegan food market, labelled as 'healthy' and 'natural'. For most of us, we have become instant gratification consumers; whatever we want it is ours, whenever we want it, it is available. A fruit all the way from the Windward Islands can be purchased here in the UK and be quickly in my bowl at home, and it can provide me with some pleasurable memories of being 'back home' in Dominica. It can become available to me within seconds of scanning my plastic card or pressing a 'place your order now' button, regardless of the fact that it may not even naturally be in season or it may have been left sprayed with chemicals in a storage factory for months.

Let's face it, the education system has inadequately prepared us for a healthy eating lifestyle because quality diets and nutrition are not part of the life-skills curriculum. Who will teach us what foods are healthy for us, which are hybrid or which are born out of a laboratory for mass consumption? Who will teach us the science of food, and how to eat well? Let us face it, do we really want to know? There may be some readers asking "What on earth has all of this got to do with fibroids anyway?"

Somewhere along the way we have lost sight of the whole purpose of food, which is to nurture and heal us, in order to have healthy, productive and purposeful lives. Nowadays, the food market is largely profit driven, and food created to satisfy our heightened pleasure-zones and our cravings for *dopamine* and the other so-called 'happy hormones', we often feel devoid of. Food can often be yet another tool that we use to buffer our feelings of powerlessness, dissatisfaction and depression, in a world which promotes apartments as opposed to homes, competitiveness as opposed to collaboration, communication and intercourse via Social Media and a disconnection with Self. All of this has taken many of us off the healing track.

So, in treating fibroid masses we need to look at the issue of food toxicity, because fibroids are created due to *toxic overload*, an *excess* of something, which then creates inflammation, energy stagnation, blood stagnation and oestrogen dominance.

It is interesting to note that fibroids are often termed the *second liver*, because our original liver, due to lifestyle choices, can become redundant in its role of effectively eliminating toxins from the body. These toxins are identified as harmful compounds by the liver, but when overloaded, it can often fail in its elimination role. Yes, this is the liver's primary job, and yet it's saying, "I cannot do this anymore!" Furthermore, the rate at which the liver can eliminate toxins is determined by a range of hereditary factors, such as our general health, our liver health, and our susceptibility to *toxic overload*. When the liver is unable to reject excess toxins, these are deposited somewhere else in the body for storage. This can eventually create masses in the lining of the uterus; this area being a safe, non-threatening environment for these fibroid masses to grow. Just look at the structural makeup of the womb; a cavity with access to a great blood supply network, which can assist a baby to thrive and grow. Well, toxins get stored there and result in the formation of fibroid masses, thriving and growing out of that rich blood supply. Ill-health ensues when the liver is unable to eliminate these toxins at the rate at which they are being introduced. For many of us we can see from the list below, the range of food we buy and eat daily which is contributing to toxic overload; white bread, margarine, jams, eggs fried in refined oils such as sunflower oil, fried bacon, coffee with dairy milk, and sugary cereals with more dairy milk, fried pork sausages, baked beans in aluminium cans…and that's just breakfast. Need I say more!

So, the fibroid becomes the *second liver*; storing toxins which were ready for the detoxification process. The only problem is that unlike the liver the fibroid cannot cleanse itself. Nature did not create the fibroid, so it does not have a self-cleansing function. It just stores the toxins and continues to grow as it gets fed with more and more oestrogen and toxins which flood our body system through our blood supply.

When we bombard our body with poor quality, processed, refined or synthetic foods, a cocktail of negative emotions, and the effects of an over-zealous lifestyle, then it is no wonder the liver gets overtaxed. We stress the liver further when we add to its already challenging role of breaking down and eliminating the biproducts of nutrients, hormones and bacterial waste from the intestines. The liver just says, "Hey! Give me a break!"

Are we getting the message? Put plain and simple, the liver goes off on holiday and starts giving up on us because we have given up on it. There is only one disease and that is toxicity. You may benefit from having a Bio Scan, a toxicity assessment which can inform you of the specific types and quantities of toxins in your system, and work from there to eliminate them. So, beloved, there is only one solution and that is to DETOX!

Oestrogen Dominance, the Endocrine System, and the Adrenals

Many of us found out about hormones from our school biology classes, where we were told about their key role in the reproductive system. To fully understand the importance of hormones, and how they function, we would need to study them further as they have an intricate purpose and value in our lives.

Hormones are chemical messengers produced by the endocrine glands, and then released into the bloodstream. They help to regulate many of the bodily functions and processes, such as sleep, appetite, and body growth. The sex hormones play a major role in sexual development, reproduction, and our general health. They are mainly produced in the ovaries, adrenal glands, and, during pregnancy, in the placenta. In women, the main sex hormones are oestrogen and progesterone, and they both play a key role in regulating bone and muscle growth, hair growth, distribution of body fat, inflammatory responses, regulation of cholesterol levels, invigorating our sexual desire and libido and much more. Testosterone is also present in women as well as men, and affects fertility, menstruation, red blood cell production, libido, tissue, and bone mass.

The metabolism of oestrogen takes place in the liver; hence we can start to make the connection between the liver's fundamental role in eliminating toxic overload, to help us address oestrogen excess which can lead to fibroids. Hormonal imbalances can be a sign of an underlying health condition, and they can also be a side effect from women taking lots of pharmaceutical drugs. When there is too much oestrogen in a woman's body and not enough progesterone, this is called oestrogen dominance, and can lead to the range of health problems listed below:

- Heavy menses
- Fibroids and cysts
- Irritability
- Anxiety and depression
- Sugar cravings
- Pre-Menstrual Symptoms (PMS)
- Headaches
- Fibrocystic breasts or swollen breasts
- Low libido
- Leg cramps
- Infertility
- Dizziness
- Water retention

Oestrogen dominance is a term used to describe a situation where a woman has an excess of oestrogen, or when she is deficient in oestrogen but has no counterbalancing hormones, such as progesterone, to mitigate the effects on her body. The increase in oestrogen dominance cases appear to be linked to the rise in environmental toxins, which introduce a vast array of oestrogen-mimicking chemicals into our environment, and our body systems. These chemicals are called xenoestrogens and can be found in many man-made compounds such as polystyrene, plastics, and household sprays. Consider tinned food which is often lined with plastics, or non-stick pans (yes, Teflon is a plastic), plastic bottles and so on. Chemicals including pesticides and insecticides which contain toxins such as Dichlorodiphenyltrichloroethane (DDT), and Polychlorinated Biphenyls (PCBs), are also known to have oestrogen-mimicking properties.

Fibroids are responsive to hormones because the fibroid tissue itself has receptor sites for oestrogen and progesterone, and a compound which mimics oestrogen would be able to enter the bloodstream, access the nucleus of the cells, dock at these receptor stations, creating cell disruption and mutation, which then leads to fibroid formation and acceleration of fibroid growth. The body's existing hormones can do their work if the body is healthy, and if there are sufficient healthy receptor sites, but what if the body is receiving oestrogen-mimicking hormones masquerading as oestrogen? Yes, I know it sounds like a Sci-Fi movie but that is something for us to marvel on later in terms of the divine intelligence creating this vessel and the world in which we live.

Our hormonal system links to the psycho-neuro-endocrine and immune systems. They are involved in an interconnected dance to maintain a balance in the mind, body, and spirit. The cell-receptors on the surface of each cell, moment to moment, send-off messages to the brain of either a *stress alarm* or *homeostasis* (peace or stability). These signals are vibrational, chemical, and hormonal, or nutritional based, and determine the amounts of hormones that get released. So, it is important to note that all sources of oestrogen, whether environmental, dietary, or endogenously produced, can and will affect fibroid growth and it is essential for these excess hormones to be eliminated.

Stress responses to life challenges can also create real physical changes in the body, and can harm the neurological, immune, and endocrine systems. The adrenals play a key part in manufacturing numerous hormones in our body and have a role in regulating the levels of minerals that our body needs. Whenever we experience a fight, flight, or freeze response to a given situation, adrenalin and cortisol flood the body system. These hormones can create havoc if they are excreted in excess and over extensive periods. A prolonged stress response, whether it be environmental, physical, or emotional, will damage the adrenals, and if the adrenals get taxed in this way, this can lead to toxic build up and adrenal exhaustion, whereby the body gives up its ability to maintain our hormonal levels efficiently. This can further lead to anxiety and other adverse effects. In the later chapters around diet and nutrition, you will note that vitamin B, vitamin C, magnesium, zinc, potassium, phenylalanine, tyrosine, and adaptogenic herbs (these counteract the effects of stress in the body), are important for hormonal health, so speak to a health practitioner for further guidance.

The thyroid regulates metabolism, and it may start to reduce its ability to balance and regulate the hormones in the body, which can then lead to cysts, fibroids, endometriosis, heavy bleeding etc. It is best to also check the levels of thyroid hormones, as these hormonal imbalances can cause oestrogen levels to become too excessive for the body to eliminate efficiently. This can then lead to fibroid masses developing in the fibrous tissue of the womb, due to the body storing this excess oestrogen.

Relative progesterone deficiency caused by chronic stress, can lead to the body getting the erroneous message that it is no longer time to procreate, and so it makes cortisol preferentially over oestrogen. Our balancing of hormones is a very delicate dance, and when there is too much oestrogen in comparison to progesterone, problems can arise. Many factors such as stress, food choices, exposure to toxins and the state of our organ functionality can all impact on our hormone levels.

Women I have worked with to eliminate their fibroid symptoms have commented how natural hormone regulators such as Maca and Vitex, and a plant-based diet, have assisted them greatly in reducing or eliminating these symptoms caused by hormonal imbalances. Supporting the parasympathetic nervous system to remain in a relaxed mode is also critical, so meditation, breath therapy, energy work, eating allergen-free and low-glycemic foods, cruciferous vegetables, and foods with high natural fats, can all contribute towards womb-wellness.

Obesity, Weight Management and Fibroids

Research shows there is a strong correlation between fibroids and obesity. This may be due to an increased conversion of oestrogen in the body's fatty tissue, when we put on weight due to fat intake and lack of exercise. One study found that there were more oestrogen and progesterone receptors in fibroid tissue than in a uterus where there were no fibroids. The xenoestrogens from environmentally toxic chemicals mentioned earlier in this chapter, also play a major role, as the liver and kidney (both critical to the detoxification process) become compromised and toxins remain stored in fat cells around the body. If the liver starts functioning poorly, then there will be excess oestrogen remaining in the blood, and the insulin which controls the blood sugar levels will be affected. This will stimulate the release of growth hormones, which in turn will increase the risk of fibroid formation and/or accelerated fibroid growth.

Many of us are eating the wrong things and at the wrong times. The acceleration of fast-food consumption, dominates our hectic lifestyle, and many women I work with complain they no longer have time to prepare their food from scratch using fresh, raw products. We are also often not mindful *how* we eat, assimilate, and digest our food and the emotional challenges affecting us affects our spleen/stomach region, leading to bloating, inflammation, flatulence, and other ailments. Let us put all our energy during mealtimes into eating and enable the mind, spirit, and body connection to take place. Other things can wait!

One mouthful of food sets off a whole chain reaction of subtle chemical processes in our mind, body and spirit, so it's important not to take food lightly. In a later chapter I mention that we have several bodies, not just the physical body, and that there are subtle substances in food which contribute to our nourishment. This can only be achieved with food that is considered 'live' or of a 'high vibration', meaning full of vital energy and nutrients. Other food termed as 'dead' food, such as processed food, heavily fried etc., are depleted in energy and nutrients, and so are not growth-enhancing or healing to us at all. Our body is a magnificent machine, and we need to live in harmony with the natural laws of the universe to heal. Yet for many of us, we just snack all day.

Consuming a lot of refined sugars can promote inflammation, and lead to weight gain. Links have been made between hormonal imbalance and weight gain, which are both causative factors of fibroid growth. High Glycaemic Index is a measure of how quickly a food causes our blood sugar levels to rise. These foods are quickly digested and absorbed and can cause a rapid rise in blood sugars. Women who eat a lot of food with a high Glycaemic Index (GI), refined sugars, fried chips, commercial breads etc., are also at risk of getting fibroids, because this can cause insulin spikes, changing hormonal levels. Many of these processed foods have been stripped of all nutrients, where only high carbohydrates are left. These are what we often term as *'empty foods'*.

Acidic Food

One example of toxicity is the acidic diet of the vast majority of the world's population. With the increased consumption of processed foods making up a large percentage of family meals these days, the content tends to be more on the acidic pH range instead of an alkaline, the latter deemed healthier. A pH of 7.0 is neutral; with 14 being the most alkaline level and 0 being the most acidic level. When we consume a heavily acidic diet, the body can react antagonistically to pH level foods lower than 6pH. There are many foods that we consume daily which may be wreaking havoc on our health, and you may be surprised to know that foods such as corn oil, white sugar, artificial sweeteners such as aspartame, mayonnaise, wheat, coffee, and processed cheese are on the acidic pH range, and too much can be very toxic for the body.

The stomach is typically pH 3.5 because of its role in breaking down food. It too has a very delicate balance which should not be tipped into excess. In trying to work more towards an alkaline diet you may want to introduce alkaline foods such as lentils, miso, tempeh, unsweetened dairy-free yoghurt, fresh vegetables, quinoa, millet, olives, peppermint tea, avocadoes, cashew nuts, and pumpkin seeds, to name a few.

When trying to eliminate fibroids, it is not helpful to eat certain foods such as grains in large quantities, as they are known to disrupt the balance of acid in the kidneys and can create mineral deficiency which can lead to a host of health problems. Grains have become part of most people's daily diet and we are eating these at a much higher rate than ever before. The agricultural revolution has made grains far more accessible now, and our bodies are just not equipped to manage the volume. Grains are complex carbohydrates that break down into sugars in the body, too much of this can significantly spike our blood sugar and insulin levels, leading to insulin resistance and toxic overload. Potato turns to sugar, yet on the average day in the UK an adult could eat chips or crisps for lunch, mash potato for dinner and more fries for evening leisure time, all soaked up with carcinogenic, acidic oils from the frying process. Most studies will show us that a pH level of 7.365 in food is quite balanced, and yet our typical diet in the UK consists primarily of foods that have an acidic range of 6-4 or below.

If we start to understand that our body, mind, and spirit are one interconnected system, then we can reason that whatever we put into that system can tilt this delicate balance, tipping it into imbalance quite easily, and often unknowingly. Our ideal blood pH level is between 7.35 and 7.45. It is noted that if we eat highly acidic foods, this can create toxins which can cause bone and muscle deterioration, as the body will extract its supply of calcium to try and restore the balance. Bones and muscle need this calcium, so become deficient and brittle when it is used for body restoration. There are many studies that link acidic food to arthritis, cancer, liver problems and heart disease, and this issue of toxins links back to the previous section about the liver's role in toxic waste elimination.

Our body needs to maintain a balanced pH level and all our cells need oxygen but yet the amount of oxygen we intake is usually inadequate and the quality poor. Body cells use oxygen to transfer energy stored in our foods into a usable form. This process allows cells to harness this energy to perform their vital functions. Oxygen is also required to build new cells and tissue, replace old tissue, dispose of waste and to reproduce new cells. Without oxygen, we would not be able to function for a long period, and if we deprive a cell of 35% of its oxygen through improper diet, incorrect breathing, and poor-quality water, over a period of time these cells can start to become cancerous. It is important for us to appreciate just how crucial diet, nutrition, correct breathing, and water are for us to maintain our pH levels.

Everything is divinely engineered to maintain balance and homeostasis, else things fall apart. The gut already has a higher acidic pH level to break down our ingested foods, and so adding high levels of acidic foods can take the gut environment into a toxic state; create allergic reactions, acid reflex disorders and more. Toxins that become excessive in our body system, can create a pathway to dis-ease; creating mucus which then leads to inflammation of the cells in the gut, colon, lungs etc.

According to Robert Young in his book *The PH Miracle: Balance Your Diet, Reclaim Your Health*, an imbalanced pH can lead to cellular interruptions, diabetes, cardiovascular problems, and cancer. It can drastically shorten our lifespan and lead to all sorts of health problems that we brush aside as 'old age'; and yet if we get the pH balance right, we would not have half the health challenges we are experiencing, as an alkaline diet is known to help neutralise bacteria and other pathogens in the body.

When we eat certain types of acidic foods (processed, animal protein and starches), mucus accumulates over the food as it travels down the digestive tracts to protect the digestive system from acid burns. Nature is a genius! The problem is that if we eat this type of food continually, the mucus build-up will lead to unwellness, allergic reactions and aging. Toxic overload WILL contribute to fibroid growth. You would be amazed just how much mucus and toxins, and how many parasites and worms, are in our body systems due to the type of food many of us are eating every day.

The more we take time to research and learn about the level of toxicity in many of the foods we eat, the more we will be able to shift and place our healing into our own hands.

I need my SUGAR!

When I was growing up in Dominica, a Caribbean island with an abundance of fresh fruit, I recall my early childhood memories visiting the local stores with my father. The stores were filled up with lots of healthy fruit and vegetables, and local produce, but my eyes were always fixed on the locally made or imported sweets and chocolates. Yes, I was one of those children who relished all sweet things, from condensed milk, frozen joy iced cones, tamarind balls laced with white sugar, sweet white bread, and many more delights. My favourite 'treat' was *tablet*, which was grated coconut cooked with heaps of brown or white sugar. It's funny now that something so laced with sugar could have a medicinal name, but it did provide me with some momentary pleasure I must admit.

Coming to the UK in the mid-1970s, there they were again, all these sugary sweets and chocolates, with a new term, *confectionary*. Supermarket owners strategically placed these in each aisle, to tempt our parents with 'one last thing'. These were my early recollections of this heavily promoted and extensively advertised, sanctioned drug. I am pretty sure many of you can testify to the urges and cravings evoked by sugary food, but have you ever likened sugar to drugs? I did not fully appreciate just how harmful and addictive sugar was until my late thirties. It certainly would have been one of the major contributors to my fibroid growth as fibroids LOVE sugar!

Sugar is one of the main causes for inflammation in our body, and over 75% of processed foods consumed daily, contain *hidden* sugars with a myriad of names such as fructose, dextrose, glucose, sucrose, etc; all stacked up in jars of sauces, breads and even in baked beans. Yes, it's a multi-billion-dollar industry keeping us all hooked. Like any business, you need to consider what keeps your customers wanting more, coming back for their repeated visits, purchases and dare I say 'hits'. Sugar creates the temporary and illusionary effect that we yearn for, this quest for 'pleasure'. The funny thing is, this pleasure principle already resides in each one of us.

The effect of sugar on the brain is also quite phenomenal, in the sense that it gives us a rush; making us want more of that 'white stuff'. Here is a list of some of the signs indicating mild to severe addiction to sugar; binging, withdrawal symptoms, cravings, and addiction transfer to other addictive substances. Do any of these sound familiar to you? Have you noticed after taking a couple of sweet biscuits, when you look down you are surprised to find the whole pack nearly gone? Or is that just me? Well, that is the sweet-stuff addiction that most of us have a 'Jones' for. Much of the contemporary diets worldwide are riddled with sugar, and yes, it does leave you wanting more! When you have a bowl of broccoli placed in front of you, do you start to salivate? When you eat a plate of broccoli, despite it being life-sustaining, do you crave to have more and more of it? Mmmm, I don't think so!

Neurotransmitters (chemical messengers in the brain) are used by the neurons to communicate and facilitate all organ activity between the brain, body, and the nervous system. These key messages transmitted include weight maintenance, sleep, water management, energy management, pain perception responses etc. Sugar can damage these neurotransmitters, and as a result, our vital organs can stop doing what they are naturally supposed to do, and that is keeping us balanced and harmonised. There are many different neurotransmitters in the brain and the ones which are impacted greatly by sugar are dopamine, serotonin, endorphins, and GABA. Some of these excite, others inhibit or sedate us, and sugar can interfere significantly with these functions.

There seems to be substantial research to show that a very high percentage of the modern, western-influenced world, who eat a basic, standard diet, suffer from neurotransmitter problems which can lead to depression, Obsessive Compulsive Disorder (OCD), obesity, Attention Deficit Hyperactivity Disorder (ADHD), migraines, chronic pains, fibromyalgia, cysts, and fibroids, Alzheimer's disease, adrenal failure, and other forms of unwellness, and the list goes on. Cut sugar out and you may well see for yourself that most of your minor or major ailments immediately go away, as some of my clients with joint pains have revealed.

The World Health Organisation (WHO) and the American Heart Association recommend that we limit our daily added sugar intake to nine teaspoons (38 grams) for men and six teaspoons (25 grams) for women. Other studies recommend that we limit our daily fructose intake to less than 25 grams from all sources, including natural sources such as fruit — regardless of whether you are male or female. That equates to just over six teaspoons of total sugar a day. Perhaps measure the sugar content in all foods eaten for a day; that exercise may surprise many of us.

Studies have shown that the average person in the UK consumes around 15-20 teaspoons of added sugar a day, which is about three times the recommended amount. There is no doubt that this over consumption of sugar is fuelling the obesity and chronic disease epidemics we are currently struggling with here in the UK.

To experience a state of well-being, all the brain chemicals need to be functioning properly, and too much sugar can cause an excess secretion of 'happy hormones', which can make us want more to satisfy ourselves and to keep that 'feel good' factor going. When we eat a lot of refined, processed sugars, they can trigger the production of the brain's natural opioids, a key ingredient in the addiction process. Our brain essentially becomes addicted to stimulating the release of its own opioids, as it would to addictive drugs like morphine and heroin.

Genetically Modified Organisms (GMOs)

Despite the nutritional guidelines to eat more fruit and vegetables, less than half a percent of agricultural subsidies go towards growing such healthy foods. According to GeneWatch UK, in 2015, GMO crops were grown in 28 countries across the world and on 179.7 million hectares of land. That is seven times the land mass of the UK. GMO crops that enter Britain are mainly used for animal feed, and we are told that none are used for commercial growing, except for some trials in GMO potatoes, wheat, and flax in recent years. We can ask the question though, what happens when GMO foods enter the blood supply of an animal fed on it, and then we eat the animal? Meat and dairy produced by animals fed on GMO foods do not have to be labelled according to EU regulations, so what does this mean for many who do not wish to have GMO foods in their food supply chain?

It is important to note that although many avoid soy because they know it to contain oestrogen-mimicking properties, more work on phyto-oestrogens needs to be done to contest this. We should also be concerned about the common meats and dairy products laden with oestrogen-mimicking properties that many in the world are eating. Many animals used for meat and dairy consumption in the food market are commonly supplemented with synthetic growth hormones. Because the cow contains its own naturally occurring oestrogen, we are getting a double dose of oestrogen when we eat conventionally farmed livestock and dairy products. This excess can lead to toxic overload in the system as the liver is trying to eliminate the excess oestrogen, at a slower rate than we keep pumping it in.

More than 50% of land in US for example is used for growing GMO soybeans and corn. Much of the corn is refined into sugar or used to feed animals that many of us eat. We are actively supporting a diet laden with sugars; mainly consisting of processed grains, namely high-fructose corn syrup (HFCS), GMO grain-fed cattle, and GMO soybean oil, all of which are now well-known contributors to obesity and chronic disease, yet because it is a highly profitable industry, you try taking it away! As these large international biotech companies aggressively promote GMO foods, because it has become a financial gold mine, there are concerns that they are linked to the promotion of abnormal cell growth, which can lead to fibroid growth.

For some of us, food was something sometimes denied to us as children, or associated with some form of punishment. For others, we use food as comfort and eat after arguments or when there is tension in our bodies and in our homes. A good friend calls it 'constant grazing'. We must ask ourselves important questions to ascertain our healthy or unhealthy emotional responses to types of food and consider some lifestyle changes if we want fibroids to shrink.

One of the choices might be to start moving towards a more plant-based diet. One way I try to remind myself of the healing properties of fresh, live, plant-based food is by observing what sunlight does to plants, and how we benefit fully from this life-sustaining quality of live food, because of solar energy shining on it and through it. This, in turn, gets transferred to us once we partake of this life-enriching food. Yes, I want some of this energy!

Growth Hormones in Meat and Dairy Products

Much of the milk sold in supermarkets comes from cows that have been treated with a synthetic growth hormone called Recombinant Bovine Growth Hormone (rBST) to make them produce more milk. Cows already have a naturally occurring form of the same growth hormone, and there are concerns about adding more into their system. These cows injected with rBST tend to also have an increase in insulin-like growth factor (1GF-1) which is known to be one of the highest risk factors associated with early puberty, breast cancers and growth formation. Yet, the media actively promotes the purchase of cow's milk and dairy products, and oftentimes parents believe this is the best way for their children to obtain calcium for bone development and maintenance. What they end up receiving are the growth hormones and other chemicals deposited into most of the world's milk. Conventional milk comes from cows that have been injected with hormones such as rBST and it cuts the cow's lifespan in half. The average glass of milk has over 20 different chemicals in it just to process it and get it in shops and into your fridge, in the name of convenience.

The growth-producing hormones being added to our food such as milk, cheese, and the finger-licking chicken, are all increasing our exposure to these environmental toxins.

To Soy or Not to Soy

In 2005 I became a vegan and started off having a close relationship with a range of soy products. In my mind, it would form the basis of my protein intake for the years to come as I removed meat and dairy products from my diet. I was elated to find a meat-substitute, and in my attempts to delight myself and the family, I soon turned my hand to jerk tofu, scrambled tofu, soy sausages, and bought soy ice-cream for dessert. I did not know then that protein could also be sourced from other foods such as quinoa, almond milk and lentils, nor did I appreciate that some of the products I ate still have a lot of GMO soy in them. What I did notice during this time was that my fibroids were growing, and they were growing at an accelerated speed as my soy intake increased.

There is a vast array of differing views and opinions about whether soy is good or bad for fibroid health and I am not able to advise whether to cut it totally out of your diet. I did find, that in keeping a journal around my dietary changes in relation to fibroid shrinking, the less soy I ate and drank, the fibroids did not get larger. On a trip to the US in 2015 where I ate tofu daily, drank soya daily and had soya in my coffee once a week, my fibroids grew double in size when I had them measured upon my return to the UK.

But soy has been a major staple diet of Asian cultures for centuries, and there is a low incidence of fibroids in those parts of the world (excluding more recent city-dwellers living a more Western diet and lifestyle). If we dig a little deeper, then we find that the root of the problem may be more in the processing of the soy for the global market leading to poor production standards and genetic modification. The misinformation about soy has led many to opt out of having it in their diet; ignoring the fact that there are rich phytoestrogens in soy products which is seen to be good for body-wellness. Good sources of soy are rich in protein, micronutrients, calcium, iron, vitamins B1, 2, 3, 5, 9, vitamin C and zinc, but it is critical that we make healthier choices to use non-GMO soy from tofu, edamame (whole soybeans) and tempeh, and only purchase reputable sources of soya milk. Perhaps also the age-old adage, "everything in moderation" serves us well in certain situations.

Many research documents assert that only fermented soy foods are safe and healthy to consume, with the eating habits of traditional Asian cultures cited as support for this claim. In fact, contrary to this common misconception, the soy products regularly consumed in Asian countries are not all, or even primarily, fermented. According to research from Ginny Messina, R.D., "In Japan, about half of soy consumption comes from the fermented foods Miso and Natto, and half comes from tofu and dried soybeans. In Shanghai, most of the soy foods consumed are unfermented, with tofu and soymilk making the biggest contributions. In Indonesia, tempeh is a well-known and revered national food, unfermented soy products like tofu account for around half of soy intake."

Today, 81% of the global soybean crop is genetically modified. The GMO soy consumed by farmed animals is one of the main sources of protein for cows. When we start to join up the dots, we can see that this soy gets retained in the milk that most people drink, or on our plates as the vast array of meat dishes people eat daily. It even gets included in some of the vegetarian or vegan products we consume. Now, ask a question, is there a correlation between the soy allergy acceleration and GMO increase? Research shows that allergies rocketed by 50% in the UK at the time when there was a huge influx of GMO soy imported from the US, flooding into the UK market.

When making your choices, I would suggest you are moderate or take it out of your diet fully and measure the impact for 6 months. It would also be advisable to buy as much locally grown, organic produce that is in season from your local Farmers' market. At least with organic foods, care and consideration is usually taken to eliminate harmful pesticides from our food chain. These harmful chemicals can seep into our fatty tissues, where they can mimic oestrogen. These oestrogen mimicking deposits can contribute to fibroid formation and the accelerated growth of cysts.

Environmental and Household Toxins

When we look at the causes of fibroids, we see that the health of an individual is evidently the consequence of the interplay and integration of two major factors: the internal environment and the external one. The external environment impacts greatly on fibroid masses on a cellular level through the exposure of heavy metals and chemicals. More general reasons for the acceleration of fibroids are linked to the vast number of harmful chemicals which are now in our day-to-day environment. As the modern world turns over billions of new products each week to fulfil our material needs, wants, and desires, we have become increasingly vulnerable to thousands of new environmental toxins. There are hundreds of harmful chemicals in the plastic and polystyrene containers we use for our food storage; chemicals such as Poly-Chlorinated Biphenyls (PCBs), Organo-Chlorines and Dioxin to name just a few. We also need to be mindful of the harm which Electro Magnetic Frequencies (EMFs) are having on our health. These electric and magnetic fields exist wherever electric current flows – in power lines, cables, residential wiring, computer gadgets, and electrical appliances.

From the amalgam fillings which are constantly seeping toxins into our mouths and into our system, the aluminium pots we cook with, the vaccines we have before we go abroad, the mercury-laden drugs from many of the pharmaceuticals, the house cleaning products, to the hair, body, and skin products we use daily, toxicity is all around!

Scientific studies show that most modern diseases can be linked to environmental toxins. These toxins can create havoc on the neurotransmitters in the brain, and can have a wide array of physical and physiological effects, such as cravings for sugar, depression, chronic fatigue etc. Our soil is contaminated with herbicides and pesticides, industrial pollutants, and heavy metals. The plants absorb these toxins and we then absorb them when we eat our fill. From our carpets to our bed pillows, we see high levels of benzene and formaldehyde which can be linked to asthma, headaches, swollen glands, fatigue and more. Phthalates are found in cosmetics, air fresheners, children's toys, paint, and perfumes and yet the standards authorities deny us the truth about the serious risks to health that such poisons pose.

According to WHO, between one million and twenty-five million people across the globe suffer from pesticide poisoning each year and an even higher number affected with symptoms which create emotional, psychological, and physiological imbalances; and many do not even know their ill health is caused by these toxins. These toxins are difficult to excrete once they enter the internal system and consequently can wreak havoc for years. I will share in later chapters which supplements and herbs assist with extracting these heavy metal pollutants from our system.

Yes, we want white, healthy teeth, so we spend our money on fluoride-based toothpastes, amalgam fillings, root canals etc. Amalgam fillings contain mercury which is a powerful neurotoxin. Check out a book *Tooth Truth* by Dr Frank Jerome if you wish to know more.

Let us also explore the water we drink or bathe in. Many of us drink water from our main tap supply, and if we do not do this, we may still wash our fruit and vegetables in tap water, or shower or bathe with it. Tap water in some parts of the world is deemed to have quite a lot of toxins, and can be contaminated with pesticides, herbicides, lead poisons and other pollutants from contraceptive pills, fertilisers etc. To add insult to injury, chlorine is then added to 'clean' the water. According to the US Council of Environmental Quality, the cancer risk among people drinking chlorinated water is 93% higher than among those who drink un-chlorinated water. When chlorine is added to water, it combines with natural compounds to form tri-halomethanes or THMs. These trigger the production of free radicals in the body, causing cell damage. Help! Is this making sense to you?

If you are a vegan like me, you may have thought this stopped a lot of toxicity from entering your body, but as you can see, food is not the only way toxins get into our body systems. It is important to realise the interconnectedness in the chain of life; the air we breathe, the water supply we drink from, the factories pumping out toxic waste that we inhale, the designer perfume we spray on our skin; all these are also ways by which toxins enter the body.

It is impossible to totally avoid environmental toxins, as we can see, they are everywhere. Nor can we live in a glass bubble. There are, however, some fundamental things we can do to reduce our exposure to toxic chemicals, and this entails making some simple lifestyle changes listed below:

- For your drinking water, buy a good quality water filter, and drink water at a pH balance of 7.4+
- Avoid storing water in plastic in the freezer or in a hot car
- Shop and eat organically
- Eat less processed foods
- Purchase an Electro Magnetic Frequency (EMF) shield to guard from environmental toxins
- Use environmentally friendly washing products for your clothes and those with the least amount of toxic chemicals. Or consider making your own
- Stop using bleached sanitary pads; use only environmentally friendly and chemical-free brands. Some women also opt for alternatives like making their own cloth pads or using menstrual cups
- Use organic cotton bedding and natural fibres
- Use environmentally friendly, ethically tested, paraben and sulfate free, non-toxic and as natural as possible, hair, body and beauty products; soap, shampoo, cream, cosmetics, perfume, deodorant etc
- Avoid deodorant containing aluminium
- Avoid toothpaste containing fluoride
- Be cognisant of the quality of air where you live and make changes if possible
- Unless filtered, avoid tap water for washing food and cooking
- Replace amalgam fillings in your teeth with enamel
- Limit your use of mobile phones or keep them on aeroplane mode often

- Use environmentally friendly, non-toxic, natural cleaning products and natural air fresheners

Our Emotions – "I'm only human after all!"

Our thoughts and our reactions to challenging events can play a pivotal role in our ability to maintain peaceful lives, and will therefore impact on the neurological, immune, and hormonal functions of the body. You may ask "what has this got to do with fibroids?" Well, negative emotions create toxins.

Emotions are made up of a thought and an energy. It is the voluntary part (the thought) that leads the involuntary part (the energy). Another way of explaining this, and so well put by Dr Tau Napata in a lecture I attended a while back, is, "…everything involuntary within us has a voluntary handle." When we start to understand this, we can learn to respond differently to life challenges, instead of believing that all emotions are natural to us and that we cannot help but express them.

Let us look at the emotion we call anger. It is worth noting that TCM recognises that anger is diagnosed as an energy imbalance. It is therefore not natural to us, so should not be left untreated. An imbalance in the liver energy system will have physiological and emotional correspondences, such as tendon tightness, over assertion, frustration, and anger; so we cannot just say that emotions are 'natural' to us. Once a health practitioner works holistically to help improve your health, you will soon appreciate that peace and joy are the only healthy states; all other emotional states lead to imbalances and can be brought into balance for our full vitality and wellness.

What is meant by an energised thought? A good example is an incident which happened to me in my early 40s, where someone called me a racist name when I was on my way home and I 'took offense' to it. That event would not have automatically created negative emotions within me if I had not first accepted the thought and given it energy, that these people were against me, and the words were offensive to me. Don't get me wrong here, racism is not something which is correct conduct, however my emotional reaction had no impact on the person changing their behaviour, but it certainly impacted on my health for days after the event took place. Yes, I saw it as 'outrageous' and a 'threat' to my well-being, and as a result, this triggered the stress response bringing up the energetic vibration of 'anger'.

You may ask, "Imani, what else *could* you have done?" Or you might say, "Sis, you had *every right* to be angry!" Well, on reflection, and with understanding of how anger works to the detriment of health and well-being, there were many other responses I could have chosen. I could have ignored the name calling and reminded myself to stay calm, and just notified the police that a racist incident had taken place. I could have ignored the name, ignored the thought and just walked on, smiling internally. I could have recited in my mind that peace is my nature, and nothing is against me and just kept walking. If there was a genuine threat to my safety, then yes, of course I would have had to have defended myself.

Ra Un Nefer Amen asserts in his book *Stress free for life*, that it is not the event in and of itself which is stressful, but our associations, images, and thoughts we have about the event. We can review our last few years of challenging situations in life to see just how many scenarios we dealt with using anger, fear, jealousy, envy, worry, grief etc. Yes, all of these emotional reactions can and will obscure our path to wellness. When we become negatively charged with emotion, we have already set negatively charged energised thoughts into motion, which create separation, disequilibrium, and imbalance in our mind, body, and spirit. Many of our lifestyle choices, and the way we handle life events, will continue to trigger this stress (*fight-or-flight*) response, and we may wish to consider attending workshops and classes to learn how Mindfulness or Meditation can help us maintain harmony and vibrate on more healthy vibrational frequencies, to stay in a healing zone. Why not look for local classes in your area or search online.

When things are small and soft, they are much easier to melt away. You can compare a cube of ice to an iceberg to get my drift. Well, we can also apply this to our emotions that are left unattended, day to day, year to year and decade to decade. These emotions, or false and rigid ideas about ourselves, others, and/or the world, can become entrenched, leading to conditioned responses. They can become what is often termed *crystallised behaviours* and get in the way of our healing process.

The Stress Response

The stress response or the *fight-or-flight* response is a physiological response that gets triggered when we experience a perceived harmful event, such as an attack or threat to our survival. With every type of stress, the trigger starts off in the hypothalamus. According to Harvard Health Medical School, a stressful situation could be environmental such as the recent COVID pandemic or psychological such as worrying about being made redundant from our job. Either way, the response triggers a cascade of stress hormones that produce physiological changes in the mind, and in the energetic and physical body. The stress response evolved as a survival mechanism that allowed us to respond quickly to a host of life-threatening situations that required us to run away or fight, and there remains a legitimate need for us to sense real danger, and to then take action. The problem with this mechanism is that it can also get triggered in day-to-day situations which are not life-threatening at all, such as disagreements in the family, being stuck on a train when there is an obstruction on the railway track, or when recalling past experiences which we labelled as 'terrible'.

This response starts in the brain when we have stressful life events. Information passes to the amygdala, a part of the brain responsible for the emotional processing of information it receives. The amygdala interprets these images and sounds received, and when it perceives danger, it immediately sends an alarm or distress signal to the hypothalamus, located in the limbic brain. This sets off the first hormonal chain reaction.

The *fight-or-flight*, or stress response, can impair the messages and commands sent out by the hypothalamus, which will have an impact on your balance and the timing of your menstrual cycles. This fight-or-flight response can also have a negative effect on the adrenal glands and its production and level of hormones such as cortisol, dehydroepiandrosterone (DHEA) and pleasure hormones. As the hypothalamus is the command centre, it communicates through the autonomic nervous system, to the rest of the body, on how to act. This nervous system controls our breath rate, blood pressure, heartbeat, blood vessel dilation and constriction, lung vessel dilation and constriction and more, and then the sympathetic nervous system triggers the fight-or-flight response, providing the body with a rush of energy to run away, fight the person, or a host of other reactions that we know so well. We now see why we get so hot and sweaty palmed just by thinking about something which was challenging to us. Try it now just for 4 seconds. Recall a situation that made you angry or scared. Did you notice any physiological changes occurring in your body?

This stimuli from these images and thoughts hit the hypothalamus, and messages get sent to the pituitary gland, which then sends signals to the thyroid gland, the adrenal gland, and the ovaries. The pituitary gland is responsible for secreting the amounts of hormones and types of hormones to the body. The levels of stress hormones such as cortisol will increase during these stress responses, and they flood the body. Cortisol can often take as long as 5 days to exit the body with each emotional episode, so we can see how too much stress can significantly affect the levels of oestrogen which gets released, disrupting the whole reproductive system and the rest of the body. Cortisol increase will cause our insulin levels to rise, so we need to also make the connection between the stress response and diabetes.

As mentioned earlier in the chapter, excess hormones can create problems when the liver is unable to play its fundamental role of detoxification, due to the bombardment of toxins it now attempts to eliminate. This can often upset the balance of Luteinizing Hormones (LH) in the body, which can then create oestrogen dominance. Oestrogen excess can affect the way in which the lining of the uterus grows and cause it to grow at an excessive rate, which then develops into fibroids.

Repeated activation of this stress response can take its toll on the body, and lead to over-toxicity. Many of us have been brought up to believe, and to accept, that negative emotions and negative emotional *reactions*, are 'natural', and there is nothing we can do to stop them. How many times have we said, "I got mad, I'm only human after all!" What if I told you that being angry is a compulsion and not a conscious choice we make, and that we can reprogramme our minds to have a different response, *react* differently to a challenging event? With practice, that different reaction then becomes our new conscious default, our new 'natural' way of responding to challenging or triggering situations.

We often fail to see the interconnectedness between ourselves and other living things, yet there is an unseen thread always working, binding us back towards peace, towards all that is natural, to a state of balance. By ensuring we are not led by our negative emotions, we can be guided to experience our true Self and our interconnectedness with all things. When we dislocate with that higher connection, we can often feel unfulfilled, dissatisfied, or empty, and this can result in us trying to satisfy our sensual urges in destructive ways. The mind evokes the thoughts around disappointment or having low self-esteem, and we then start to feel that low, and act out of that feeling. In the same way, we can accept positive thoughts about ourselves and life generally, which will, in turn, affect how we feel and act.

Suppression and Pushing Down Trauma

The body truly has the capacity to heal itself, and when we take allopathic drugs, these often push the disease deeper into the body-system, into the organs. Emotional trauma can cause a great deal of pain if the issues are not worked through in some way, whether through creativity, self-help, a health professional or some other healing process. Pain is a side effect of the body getting rid of toxins. The body is a living organism, and it will intuitively react to combat any toxins it detects in the body, and yet many of us will take pharmaceutical drugs to get rid of the pain, but the real issue and source of the problem remains masked. I would question if many allopathic drugs have qualities to heal, without creating other side effects and long-term unwellness.

We can explore fibroids using a homeopathic framework, where a homeopathic practitioner can look at the emotional, mental, psychological, and spiritual well-being of their patient. Here, a good friend of mine and excellent practitioner introduced the term *miasm* when working to assist women with fibroids. Miasms are any toxic or noxious influence on the body, producing illness, and fibroids and cysts sit within this miasm characterisation in homeopathy, due to the fact that these conditions are linked to growths caused by an excess state, and are often denoted by an over functioning, *hyper*, system.

With fibroids we see there is an over-production of something, an excess of something, bringing about pathological changes in the uterus, leading to the formation of these masses. As discussed earlier, research shows that fibroids are linked to oestrogen dominance (excess). Fundamentally, miasms are mainly caused by suppression, so homeopathic practitioners look at the multi-layers of a woman's life, and in the context of the multi-suppressors experienced by her, in order to get to the source of the condition.

A key feature of a miasm is conscious or unconscious suppression and when treating an illness or a psychotic miasm, the therapist would look at the way in which we as women suppress things, hold things in, and hold on to things.

A calcification of a fibroid would immediately alert us to the fact that there is a pattern of excess here, and that the liver, with its major role of detoxification, has been obstructed in eliminating excess toxins. So, in its inability to get rid of the excess calcium in this case, it retains it and a hardened shell is formed around the fibroid.

Take time to reflect on the things we hold on to that we should shed. What are the things we are suppressing? What are the things we are dissatisfied about? What do we crave and long for with a sense of great unfulfillment? What are we excessively thinking about, or excessively doing which is causing such disturbances in our internal environment? Joy is one of the most healing emotions we can experience. Make time to schedule in healthy activities which help invoke the joy faculty within and where there is past trauma, I encourage seeking professional help to work through this and fly!

CHAPTER 4
Black Women and Fibroids

I dedicate this chapter of the book to the specific needs of Black women who have, or are experiencing fibroids, sharing my personal journey, and the narratives of many other women who came together to heal, to address the gross disparities of fibroid growth and acceleration across the globe.

Black women are profiled as one of the highest groups with fibroids; 3-6 times more likely, and in many cases, to have multiple and larger growths. In my work as a holistic health practitioner, I am starting to see an increase of fibroid cases amongst younger Black women, and further research needs to be done to examine the reasons for this spike. There are also growing concerns that when fibroids are meant to decrease in size during the menopausal stage, for many Black women, they are not shrinking.

UK research cited that 55% of Black women will develop fibroids during their life, and the majority felt that they did not receive quality precautionary guidance or information about the full range of conventional and holistic treatment options available to them. It would be a whole new book to look at all the differences for Black women which make us more prone to fibroids, much of this relates to the higher sulpheric content in melanated people, which means our experience is significantly different to white people, and thus treatments must take ethnicity into consideration as our bio-chemistry differs. When we look at the rising statistics for Black women with fibroids, it becomes obvious that we urgently need to make more demands for specific research to be undertaken.

More research also needs to be undertaken to ascertain why Black women are known to develop fibroids at a much earlier age, and with a higher frequency compared to other ethnic groups. Recent research highlighted strikingly higher levels of aromatase located in the fibroid cells of African-American women, compared to white and oriental women in the US. (African-American 83 fold, Caucasian-American 38 fold, and Japanese 33 fold). Aromatase mRNA is the key enzyme for oestrogen production and an excess of this enzyme can lead to elevated tissue concentrations of oestrogen. It is found in the ovaries, adrenal glands, the placenta, and other reproductive areas, and we need to establish what is leading to this excess in Black women, contributing to fibroid formation and accelerated growth. Further research will help ascertain the underlying causes and what natural treatments can be administered to reduce aromatase levels in the body when in excess, and inhibit the excess production in the first place.

But we can begin by looking at the historical journey of Black women, to explore why our shared history of enslavement, colonialism and neo-colonialism, our lived experience of oppression, discrimination, and systemic racism, creates gross health inequalities, leading to a major health crisis across the globe.

Ideological and Systemic Racism

Despite race being a social construct, racism has a very real, insidious and devastating impact on the lives of Black individuals, groups, communities and countries around the world. The African Holocaust (*Maafa*), is the most horrific, brutal and barbaric continuing tragedy in history; the total denigration of a race of people purely based on the colour of their skin, leaving a global legacy of systematic and systemic discrimination and oppression, which will take many more years of dedicated and continuous effort to eradicate.

The enslavement and displacement of Black Africans has left our communities with physical, emotional, psychological, cultural and psychical wounds, which remain unhealed and still very much with us today.

Post Traumatic Slave Syndrome (PTSS), a term coined by internationally renowned researcher Joy DeGruy, PhD, is a condition that exists as a consequence of this multigenerational oppression of Africans and their descendants, due to the continuing traumatic effects of the Maafa. Many scientists have confirmed that trauma is stored in the DNA, in the memory codes, and PTSS is identified as an underlying cause as to why many people of African origin display symptoms of Post Traumatic Stress Disorder (PTSD); largely going unaddressed, undiagnosed and untreated. We can refer to the suppression of trauma which was covered earlier, to see how this can severely impact health in a myriad of ways.

The damaging effects of the Maafa continue to be passed down through the generations, reaching into the lives of great, great grandchildren, as we have been wrenched from home and heritage; we have been severed from the very roots of our tree of life and yet we wonder why we are disproportionately represented in every health, education, and social statistic. It has impacted us in every aspect of life activity, whether it be religion, education, economics, relationships, politics, wealth, health, and identity.

There has been, and continues to be, immense harm caused to Africans across the Diaspora and we must now set about creating a new and healing paradigm shift. Most of our social structures across the Diaspora, including many countries of the African continent and the Caribbean, are also riddled with the same residual diseases of colonialism, capitalism and racist infrastructures. What was the binding glue which once kept our African nations strong for thousands and thousands of years, prior to it being dismantled? We can look at Ra Un Nefer Amen's work as a key?

I get a 'wake-up call' whenever I walk around my little country town thinking things have changed, only to then be faced with the stark reality that they have not. In my previous consultancy role, delivering Race Hate Crime Awareness training, I heard accounts from African Muslim women being spat at and taunted as they walked their children to school, or Black men at work who experienced white colleagues writing "nigger go back to your own country" on papers slipped under the cracks of their lockers. I know from my own experiences, that when there is an innate urge to unify and to be loved and accepted, the mind and body is damaged when people treat you with such disdain. It impacts greatly on maintaining a positive sense of identity and hinders many of us Black women from feeling we can be our true and authentic selves, in all our myriad skin tones, in environments which are so toxic.

Yes, racism in its varied forms, is still with us and is still embedded in the fabric of all social activity. This subject is a whole book in itself, and so I will not be able to go into much depth; however, as a Black woman, and for many other Black women, we cannot separate this shared, lived experience, from how we have learnt to view ourselves; how we feel about ourselves, and where we position ourselves (or are positioned) in the world.

In the UK, a significant number of Black women I have supported as a community leader and health practitioner over the last 25 years, have shared experiences of overt and covert racial discrimination, as well as how this impacted their health and well-being. Many did not feel that their physical environments were conducive to maintaining full health and vitality. There was a strong sense of cultural dislocation, and despite the fact that many Black women were born in the UK, or spent most of their lives in the UK, there was still a sense of "you don't belong."

In 2019/20, police crime records showed that there were 105,090 cases of race hate crime in the UK, which was 8% higher than the previous year (*commonslibrary.parliament.uk*). With the 2020 Black Lives Matter incidents, triggered by the brutal murder of George Floyd, the world became more cognisant of what had always been there; racial stereotyping, discrimination, and racially motivated murders. All these things further compound the challenges faced by Black women, and impact and trigger the stress response. Even as I sit here writing, I think of an informal support meeting booked this evening with a young Black student at the University where I live, who has asked for support due to the level of racial discrimination she is going through with a teacher on her Degree course.

This global system of racism, which constantly attempts to silence, suppress, distort the truth of who we are as a Black people, the impact of our physical, emotional and spiritual dislocation from our Motherland, cannot be spoken about enough as a way to aid healing and invoke reparation. As author Dr Lashonda M. Jackson-Dean puts it in her book *Seed to Seeds*, the "…Black race has traded the chains for handcuffs, the stowed ship undercarriage has become the police cars. The plantation is now the prison yards."

The daily bombardment of racist images, words, and aggression, constantly reminding us of our 'otherness', is not an easy road to travel, and many times, especially as women, we feel forced or manipulated to change our authentic appearance; to change our hair, our clothing, and sometimes even the colour of our skin, to try to become more acceptable; to integrate, or worse still, assimilate or blend in. It is important to recognise that the moment we do this, instead of affirming our rich African heritage and legacy, aspects of ourselves cannot be voiced, pieces of who we are get suppressed and rejected. What words do we digest and start to believe about ourselves? "I'm not light enough", "I'm not dark enough", "I wish I was like…", "I'm ugly", "I have bad hair", and other such denigrating and belittling remarks. So, what words *should* we instead tell ourselves daily, to counteract this attack on our very identity?

We cannot ignore the fact that Black women across the globe are still affected by many of these psycho-social issues. The systemic and systematic ways in which racism and sexism operates, can often make us feel that we need to deny both our femininity and our Blackness, in order to fit in, be safe, be heard, or be accepted. Black culture, use of our Black symbolism and artistic reference such as music, writing and theatre, can all play a part in imbibing a strong sense of Black identity and pride back into our psyche. So as not to adversely impact our health, we must be mindful of the thoughts we accept, and work towards affirming the true, authentic, beautiful selves that we are, instead of holding onto toxic and negatively charged ideas based on the lies we are told, and the lies we tell ourselves about who we are as a people.

As part of our healing, the issue of reparations is of major importance, but there is much we can do to heal from the psychological trauma while demanding reparations. To minimise the negative energy and tension racism and internalised racism can evoke, we can look to channelling our energies towards collective healing; start projecting images and narratives we want to see in the world; research and disseminate images which celebrate our rich heritage and our diverse culture. This paradigm shift comes by first creating an environment where healing waters can run free; where energies can be unblocked and new, surging energy can course through our veins.

Many Black women I interviewed felt that they were not able to fully express aspects of their Black culture and traditions living in the UK, even though there were many aspects about life in the UK that they enjoyed. One thing that emerged as a universal need, was for Black women to get together to experience a safe space; in order to explore how issues around health and well-being, shaped within a cultural context, affected them; to enable them to flex and be real. This was the primary reason why the Black Sister's WombWellness support circles were birthed.

Like many women across all cultural groups, there were also challenges of navigating family needs, extended family needs, relationships and family responsibilities, which often left them feeling exhausted, with little time and space to repair and heal.

Combat Fatigue – "I am tired of playing Cultural Expert"

I came across the term *Combat Fatigue* in my mid-twenties whilst working as a community officer. It is regarded as a career related syndrome, brought about by the impact of Post Traumatic Slave Syndrome (PTSS); where over time as Black people we accept and internalise the negative projections of ideas and images about our people, onto ourselves. This can often lead us to go along with the racist values, ideologies and behaviours, in ways which are internally incongruent, leading then to internal and external stress. This type of fatigue is brought about by the psychological and emotional exhaustion that many Black people experience, when in a workplace where they are in the minority, and have to constantly defend or *fight* for their rights and protect their cultural expression.

Combat fatigue can also be brought about by taking on over and above your job roles and duties; always feeling you have to please or do exceptionally well or better that your white colleagues. In addition, it can occur as a result of accepting the role of 'cultural expert' or the 'cultural font of all knowledge' in the workplace, around anything related to Equality and Diversity, as if this should not be something all staff should be committed to.

We need to stop playing cultural expert. We are often expected to come up with answers and solutions for the whole of the Black race, or come up with solutions to eradicate racism. When there is a crime committed by a white man, do you think the whole white community starts to feel collective guilt, or ashamed because of this act? The system of racism has created an innate sense of 'centrality' in the world; where being white becomes the default *central* position, and everyone else is 'other'. When there is a mugging and a Black person finds out it is a Black person who was responsible, we can often internalise feelings of shame, blame, disgust, and feel we have to apologise for it, when we did not even know the person. We feel collective trauma, and we can often feel collective fear of the repercussions when anyone in our ethnic group does wrong. No, it was not your fault, so don't carry it! Yes, offer resources and information when white colleagues want to know more about Black culture or say things which are stereotypical and need to be corrected and guided, but do not feel you have to take on the world or more than your fair share.

Examples have been shared in support groups where Black women had white people touching their hair without seeking permission, they are wearing lovely 'costumes' or saying racist statements, "but you're not like the others." In extreme cases, combat fatigue itself as having to feel we have to change our names, change our hairstyles, change our shade, to appear more 'western'; to try and assimilate and be 'approved' in the workplace. These experiences can create a great deal of additional stress on top of the usual work-related issues people have to deal with and respond to, and clients have shared symptoms such as depression, low energy, isolation, over-defensiveness, anxiety, and stress as a result.

There are times when we feed ourselves untruths and accept thoughts such as, "I am not good enough", "I am not light enough", "I cannot be successful", "I have to work 10 times as hard to get somewhere in life". Are we ourselves reinforcing negative stereotypes about us as a people? e.g. using words like nappy head, half-caste, coolie, good hair, and bad hair. How do we act in our own peer group and does this change when amongst white peers? This can be termed *cultural switching*, which may be fine, but which can be exhausting and self-destructive if we are suppressing our true selves and just behaving in a certain way to please others or to fit in, to assimilate and be 'accepted'. We have been socialised to believe that we have to change the way we inherently are, in order to fit in and this is neither true or healthy.

Through such life experiences we should remind ourselves that experiences and events are neither inherently good nor bad. When we use these labels to degrade ourselves or others, we are assigning and directing an energetic vibration, and reinforcing negative thoughts and feelings, giving energy to grow or feed fibroids. All these scripts work against our true nature, which is peace itself, and will create an imbalance or an excess (over production of toxins), within our internal system.

By learning more about our rich history and legacy that goes way back, over six thousand years of African kingship, queenship and leadership, we can use this knowledge as a compass to navigate the storms of racism and colonialism; to be able to respond from a place of peace, feeling anchored and resilient to stay well. Racism is not *our* sickness, despite us feeling the effects of it daily.

Black Hair Relaxers

There has been some research undertaken to examine whether the chemical components of leading hair relaxers can be attributed to over-toxicity and to the growth and acceleration of fibroids, particularly amongst young Black women. But even though there has not been enough extensive research to quantify this hypothesis, we can however research and learn about toxicity generally, and how it enters our body system, to form our own educated conclusions without waiting for this research to materialise.

In 2009, *Essence magazine* published an article on fibroids, and highlighted findings that in the US, fibroids grew at a 3-5 times higher rate amongst Black women who used chemical relaxers. This was further supported by another study in the American Journal of Epidemiology, where they made a connection between hair relaxers and fibroid formation and growth, as well as spurts of early puberty amongst Black young girls. During this study, they followed 23,000 pre-menstrual Black girls into adulthood, between the years 1997 to 2009, and found that fibroids grew at a 3-5 times higher rate. Scientists linked this increase to high chemical exposure through scalp legions and burns.

It is important to note that the hair care industry is not regulated by the Food and Drugs Administration (FDA), so there are no baseline standards companies have to follow to regulate the level of harm caused by such hair products. There is a deluge of hair products on the market used by the Black community. We do not need an extensive body of research to stop using these harmful chemicals and to make healthier choices. Will we wait until science categorically tells us the harm that anything toxic going into our bloodstream can cause? Let us get it straight, all relaxers and perm products are harmful to us, period! The skin breathes and pores take in toxic chemicals straight into the bloodstream.

Many of these hair products contain harmful chemicals such as sulphates which can strip our natural hair of essential oils. Parabens also are harmful chemicals, used as a preservative in many skin and hair products and are known to cause endocrine disruption, which can lead to fibroids and other hormone related conditions. Silicones are not natural hair sealants. Yes, they can give the hair a nice shine, but plastics, as mentioned before, can be harmful to our health. Phthalates are also harmful chemicals that we should avoid as they too have been linked to endocrine disruption and over toxicity. Hair relaxers include agents like Formaldehyde and Sodium Hydroxide. Formaldehyde mimics the properties of oestrogen, and this may be a contributory factor setting off hormonal imbalances, causing fibroids to grow at a higher rate and triggering a progression towards dis-ease due to toxin absorption. These toxic chemicals have direct access to our bloodstream through the skin. To heighten the impact further, they can enter at a faster rate through the legions and burns brought about by using such harsh chemicals.

CHAPTER 5
My Work with Black Women with Fibroids

Over the years many women have shared their fibroid stories with me and I formally interviewed 25 Black women from the UK and the Caribbean, as part of the initial research for this book. In this chapter I outline some of my findings.

80% of the women who attended my fibroids support groups did not feel they received adequate guidance and support from their health practitioners. 70% of Black women were strongly advised to have a hysterectomy as the primary option available to them.

Many Black women interviewed felt they submitted to the doctor's advice about the hysterectomy, because they really did not know what other options were available, and despite the vast majority preferring a non-invasive route, none were offered.

There were mixed responses in terms of the actual experience of their initial visit to the GP for checks. Some felt that they were listened to and supported, and 40% felt they had a poor healthcare service, due to feelings of being rushed and not having ample time to talk through what they were going through; particularly how the symptoms were impacting on their well-being and day to day family and work life.

These findings appear to follow similar themes across the UK, the Caribbean, and the US; where studies in the US by Dr Scott Goodwin MD found that as many as 77% of women had fibroids, and 14% of women met no valid medical criteria for undergoing the hysterectomies they were advised to undergo.

A resounding cry out from the women, was that there appears to be some 'watch and wait' advice being given upon early detection. They were not given any advice on ways to shrink or prevent fibroid growth and acceleration. The GPs suggested that they would monitor the growth pattern every 6 months or so through ultrasound. In one case 16 fibroids were removed, some had grown to the size of large oranges. This 'watch and wait' approach in my view is not advisable, as it is far easier to eliminate fibroids at an early stage when they are small, soft, and moveable, than when they have enlarged and have become calcified.

For the majority, their fibroids were first noticed through self-examination or an examination at their local clinic where they felt hard lumps rising from the surface of the skin. Most of the women spoke about their initial worry, anxiety, and feelings of isolation at this time. Many of the women had painful and increased menses much earlier on, but did not attribute it to a possible fibroid growth. Many were reluctant to share with family and friends, even after the diagnosis, and even after being told they were benign. Some did not feel able to share this with their partners and this often led to tensions in their relationships.

A small minority (2%) stated they had no symptoms or complications at all. 80% of the women became aware of their fibroid(s) late in the development of the masses despite having early symptoms which could have been detected and diagnosed as possible fibroids. The fibroids had already grown to sizes between 3-8cms by the time they went for a check-up.

20% of the women shared that their sex lives had been significantly disrupted due to heavy and prolonged menses, or that having intercourse was abandoned as it was "far too painful". In some cases, this put a great deal of strain on their relationships and some women did not feel able to share what they were going through with their partners, due to the fear of them leaving or having sex elsewhere. This further compounded their situation.

At this stage, questions may have started to form in your mind as to why, in so many cases, were the fibroids left un-treated by GPs? What was clear was that for most women I interviewed, there was a level of 'inaction' amongst health practitioners during the early stage of detection. There is still not enough known in the conventional medical arena about fibroids and their formation, and so, GPs seldom know how best to advise their patients about anything other than allopathic drugs (mainstream pharmaceuticals as opposed to homeopathic or herbal treatments), or invasive treatments. These approaches can often attempt to address the symptom without getting to the cause, and this is the reason why in many cases, the fibroids just keep on growing, or why after surgery they return.

Table: Research - 25 Black women living in the Caribbean and the UK

Themes covered	Findings
Age	• Between 40-60
Ethnicity	• African Caribbean and Black African
Work and family responsibilities	• 80% had demanding jobs • 80% had children • 10% did not have children but did have other taxing caring responsibilities in their family • Employment ranged from: Teaching in Schools, Adult Social Care managers, Computer and Business Consultants, Managers, Dance therapist/Psychotherapists. • 10% were Full-Time Students and/or Unemployed
The time of fibroid detection	• 20% had early detections from ultrasounds when fibroids were between 1-3cm in size. All were told there was no need for any treatment, and it was nothing to worry about. • 80% had late detections from ultrasounds when fibroids were between 3-8cms in size. The majority were only offered myomectomy or hysterectomy.
Single or Multiple fibroid growth	• 80% had multiple fibroids found by ultrasound scans at later stage of detection
Treatment recommended by GP (when fibroids grew larger)	• 40% Myomectomy (3-8cm multiple fibroids) • 70% Hysterectomy (all others) * Due to hysterectomy being required as fibroids grew back after myomectomy

Themes covered	Findings
Experience of healthcare options	- 80% felt that initial care during the ultrasound was good to excellent - 90% felt that the information they received about the options was limited - 90% were not informed about holistic or complementary therapies/treatments available, nor were they referred when they asked
Action taken as a result of the outcome	- The majority took action to undertake their own research online because of the limited information received. - The majority decided to change their diet by cutting out dairy or reducing red meat intake. Some started to look for alternative therapists and explore natural remedies to eliminate the symptoms or to reduce/eliminate the fibroids.
Effects on personal life	- 90% of women felt that fibroids impacted on their life and disrupted both home and working life. Some felt that it affected their relationships and their sex lives; particularly putting a strain on relationships. Menses became painful, heavy, or irregular, and there were signs of hormonal imbalance and discomfort. Low body-image was also experienced due to how clothes fitted once the fibroids grew.

In the UK, there is a 20% difference between Black patients and their white counterparts in terms of hysterectomies having to be applied due to fibroid complications. UK research undertaken between 2013 and 2015 showed that Black women felt that the treatments offered to them from mainstream health practitioners were 'limited' as they were only informed about invasive treatments such as myomectomies and hysterectomies.

In 2009, a study in the American journal of public health examined 1,863 women and found that 78% of the women having hysterectomies were Black (of African American origin). It was noted that some of the reasons for such a discrepancy were largely due to Black women having less access to information about alternative treatments; they often received inadequate health care, experienced racial stereotyping when trying to access healthcare services, and often had poor relationship with their GPs. More research will need to be undertaken around this theme in the UK.

Research also tells us that white women tend to have more available income and tend to spend more of their available income on health treatments, health supplements, relaxing holidays, stress eradication programmes and activities. Many Black women are part of an extended family and there are more demands on their income from family responsibilities. There are a range of socio-economic factors which contribute to this difference, which in many ways impact why Black women don't invest more on their personal health needs.

CHAPTER 6
Conventional Treatments for Fibroids

The treatment of fibroids is often ignored by the orthodox medical profession until much later in the fibroid growth stage. This is a cause for concern, as this can often mean the fibroid has become calcified and much harder to treat using non-surgical methods. If they have been left to increase to such a large size and number, many women often feel they have no choice but to have invasive surgery.

Hysterectomy

This is one of the most invasive treatments for symptomatic fibroids (meaning fibroids presenting with symptoms), and involves taking out the womb and oftentimes, taking out the ovaries. It is becoming far less popular now that other treatments are available to women, however, in my view, there are still very high numbers of such an invasive operation being undertaken in the UK and US.

In the UK, about 20,000 procedures are performed each year, despite there being alternative treatments available. A recent report undertaken by the *All-Party Parliamentary group on Women's health (WHAPPG)*, raised concerns about the standards of care offered to women with fibroids, where 43% of women were noted to be unsatisfied with the information received about the range of treatment options, and 67% of Primary Care Trusts were said to take little or no measures to ensure women had all the choices made available to them.

Many physicians I have spoken to believe that having this surgery has minimal long-term risks, however in my view, and from some of the research undertaken over the years, this is not the case.

Studies undertaken in the US highlighted that this operation made women more at risk to degenerative disease; they had 14% higher risk of abnormal fat levels, 13% higher risk of high blood pressure, 18% higher risk of obesity, and 33% higher risk of heart disease. There were also health concerns for women having hysterectomies when under 35 years old, where they were more at risk for congestive heart failure, and 2.5-fold greater risk of coronary artery disease due to plaque build-up in the arteries. There is also a 60% risk of urinary incontinence and an induction of premature menopause. After having this operation, there is usually a sudden drop in oestrogen and progesterone levels, which can lead to vaginal dryness and early signs of menopause such as hot flashes. Other post hysterectomy complications could include severe bleeding, vaginal vault prolapse, impaired bladder functions, lowered libido, and negative emotional and psychological effects.

Many women I have worked with who had hysterectomies because of fibroids, shared some of the side effects of this operation; such as low libido, weakness, fatigue, thyroid problems and some of these may be linked to the diminution of testosterone in their system due to the womb extraction. The roles that testosterone and Docosahexaenoic Acid ethyl ester (DHA-EE) play in a woman's life is important, as they maintain the balancing of hormones, energy levels and have anti-aging properties. Testosterone can also play a part in toning up or building up the muscle and bone structure of women and protects our levels of libido and inner core strength.

Some physicians are urging women to seriously consider non-invasive options before making the decision to have a hysterectomy, and others I have spoken to, and in my own experience, advise hysterectomy as their default. It is a big decision, as not only do hysterectomies rob us of our ability to have children, but the psychological effects can also leave us feeling a deep sense of loss and regret. All the above factors and options need to be taken into consideration and should be discussed by your physician, prior to you making your choice, but ensure you have all the information and have weighed up the pros and cons.

Myomectomy

This is still major surgery, whereby the fibroids are individually removed, and the uterus is preserved and/or re-constructed. A significant number of women who have been referred to me were considering this option as it did not seem to interfere with their ability to conceive. None the less, this is still an invasive operation, and the risks highlighted by physicians are that it can lead to excessive blood loss, torn uterine lining, infections, and bowel perforation. The uterus is weakened by this procedure, and so caesarean is often advised for future childbirth. C-Sections are known to aggravate the hormonal balance in the body, leading to further negative health symptoms.

There has been some new research conducted by the National Institute for Health Research published in July 2020 in the UK which may assist women to make more informed decisions about the treatment of uterine fibroids. During this study, 254 women took part in the trial, and researchers compared two competing fibroid treatments which present more likelihood for fertility, to see which option best reduced symptoms and improved the patient's quality of life. The results were published in the New England Journal of Medicine and showed that myomectomy resulted in a small but significantly higher quality of life compared to the Uterine Artery Embolisation.

Both UK and US research show that this is the preferred option for many women to a hysterectomy, and of the women undergoing this surgery, a review of published data found that the pregnancy rate was 40-60%; with the majority of those women being able to conceive within their first year.
It is important to note though, that 20-25% of women still ended up having a hysterectomy after the myomectomy, due to the re-emergence of symptomatic fibroids in an around the surrounding area, alerting us that the source of the problem was still left untreated.

Uterine Artery Embolization (UAE)

This is a relatively new procedure for the treatment of fibroids which became available in the mid-1990s. This is seen as non-surgical intervention and allows the uterus to remain intact. The procedure is performed by an interventional radiologist with the patient being under moderate sedation. It involves blocking the arteries that supply blood to the fibroid, with the use of a catheter. Contrast dye is injected first, to help visualise the uterine artery and the branching vessels, and then small, synthetic plastic particles are passed to the arteries via the femoral artery in the groin area. These particles are Trisacryl Gelatin microspheres and Polyvinyl Alcohol particles (a plastic that resembles coarse sand). I have been told that these are harmless, and that they cannot block other vessels around the body because they cannot be dissolved. More research will need to be undertaken as to the long-term impact of plastics in the body. Despite physicians commenting that they do not cause inflammation or allergic reactions, there are two women who have been referred to me with severe inflammation of the pelvis, resulting from having this operation.

The fibroids eventually start to shrink due to blocking the blood vessels which feed the uterus and feed the fibroid. Arterial blood can still flow to the uterus and as mentioned, we are told these particles cannot flow to other parts of the body to cause blockages elsewhere. The procedure can take about 1-2hrs.

This is becoming a popular treatment for many women with fibroids, however there are still some levels of risk such as infections, damage to other organs, severe inflammation, and pain. Many women have been able to conceive after a year of treatment, and many lead normal, pain-free lives.

Magnetic Resonance Imaging (MRI) and Other Treatments

More recent treatment developments in the medical world include Cryomyolysis where liquid nitrogen is used to freeze the fibroid and make it shrink, Laser Myolysis, Electromyolysis, where electrical currents are used to destroy the fibroid and shrink the blood vessels which feed it and Magnetic Resonance Imaging (MRI), where high vibrational ultrasound waves are used to break up the fibroid. These treatments are deemed non-invasive. They are outpatient procedures with decreased bleeding and decreased long-term symptoms such as pelvic pressure, inflammation, and pain. However, they are all relatively new procedures and there is insufficient research to show success rates and one's ability to conceive post-treatment.

Drug Treatments

Gonadotropin-Releasing Hormone (GnRH) Agonists such a *Luprolide* are often used to shrink fibroids. These are anti-inflammatory drugs in contraceptives containing oestrogen and progestin, a synthetic progestogen, and they are often offered to women in the physician's attempt to control the heavy bleeding experienced by women with fibroids, or to shrink the fibroids pre-surgery. However, there are mixed results about taking these drugs, and many of my clients have shared that the fibroids started growing back as soon as they stopped taking the medication due to side-effects. Some of the side effects include hot flashes, headaches, osteoporosis, mood changes, ovarian cysts, and weight gain. It is known that these drugs can shrink fibroids, however the oestrogen in contraceptive pills can often contribute towards their growth and acceleration of growth because of the high level of toxicity when using pharmaceutical suppressants.

Conventional strategies are not the primary solution, and physicians do not always seem to consider the connection between mind, body, and spirit. All of the above treatments, although options to consider for women, do not work towards addressing the root cause of fibroids in the first place; do not get to the root of the problem. What is causing the fibroids in the first place, and that is oestrogen excess and toxicity.

By understanding that fibroid masses are one of the body's many alarm bells ringing loudly to inform us that our internal environment is under attack from excess toxins, we can then start to appreciate that these masses are a biproduct of a mind, body and spirit which has moved away from its centre, away from a state of balance. Like all other illnesses, in our acknowledgement of this, we kick-start the healing process by first being determined to get back to the centre.

In selecting the best treatment there are many factors you would need to explore with your health practitioner; primarily, the fibroid size, the length of time you have had the fibroids, and its location in and around the womb. There are other considerations around your receptivity to non-invasive or invasive treatments, your views and feelings around holistic and alternative methods and conventional approaches, your cultural and spiritual values, and attitudes around womb removal, to name a few.

CHAPTER 7

Holistic Approaches to Fibroid Elimination

Creating a Feminine Internal Environment

So, what is this feminine internal environment? It is one that is in harmony with nature and natural vibrational frequencies. It is one which is composed of mainly yin, watery, cool, and moist energies/properties. It is one which nourishes and maintains our physiological, emotional, mental, and spiritual make-up and allows the Self to be placed at the centre of our lives as opposed to the material/physical part of us, thereby allowing us to flow harmoniously through life and all interactions. This state of peace is to guide our thoughts, feelings, choices, and actions. It is a state of coolness, relaxation, flexibility, and adaptability; a state where life is 'easy'.

In Kamitic (ancient Egyptian) history, women were the custodians of culture and spirituality due to our moist, watery nature. Our ability to retain water allows us to go into deep meditative trance and bring down spiritual insights and messages for the community about family, healing, and nation building. In this modern day living, women are drying out. By this I mean that our physiology and our temperament can become hot and dry by a range of lifestyle choices and when we get too externalised without making time to go within. We are cultivated to go out and earn a living, and there are no spiritual systems available to the masses to guide them as to what careers best suit their physiology and temperament. In a world where many women feel they are over-working, juggling a life of employment, voluntary work, home, family, and relationships, if we do not make time to heal, the odds will be stacked up against us maintaining a healthy lifestyle.

What impact does this heated up inner environment have on our feminine energy, our wellness, and our wombs? When we look at a hot and dry temperament which is by its very nature, externalised, defensive, combative, and competitive, we can see that it is heating us up too much if we do not have daily rituals to maintain that *yin* balance, and a cooler energy.

Many women are faced with challenges in life which often create a combative and competitive temperament and we are often not taught how to harmonise these hot and cool, moist and dry energies for health and longevity. In TCM, a practitioner would say that fibroids are the symptoms often caused by a body that is experiencing heat excess, so how are we going to stay in that cool, moist place which nourishes the feminine aspect of us?

Like men, we women, also need to consider how our emotions, our lifestyle activities and household gadgets, are constantly altering our vibrational frequencies; microwaves, laptops, fax machines, mobile phones, excessive bodywork training and anger, are all ways which we can get heated up daily. I invite you here to take 5 minutes to jot down the many things in your life that get you 'heated up'. Do this now, and see your body start to change and get warmed up, then heated just thinking about them. Get connected with this heat that gets raised every time we get combative or see things as antagonistic to us.

The most powerful and impactful quality to own is self-love, and then applying gratitude and appreciation to our lives. Once we start to cultivate this love and appreciation, we slowly start to get rid of that inner critic which is constantly chatting in our ear. There are many things daily that we can be thankful for, no matter how small, and yet from the many women I have been blessed to work with, I can see that we carry a lot of blame, shame and criticism for ourselves, our relationships, our children, our partners, our family, our friends, others in our community, work colleagues etc. All of this takes energy, and all of this creates tension. We need to harbour this energy and direct it instead towards our visualisations and goals, for them to come to fruition.

So, in the process of healing, we need to work on these issues and start creating a harmonious environment which initiates a healing paradigm. It starts with loving ourselves, accepting the core of who we are and knowing that we are divinely gifted and blessed and that we are not victims. If we hold on to any thoughts which do not reflect that true nature, dis-ease will be triggered. It starts with us taking ourselves away from the inner and outer noise, and allowing peace, self-acceptance, love, and gratitude to come to the fore. I have detailed some of the other practical steps for consideration in later chapters.

Traditional Chinese Medicine (TCM)

*"Nothing under Heaven is more yielding than water.
But when it attacks things hard and resistant,
There is not one of them that can prevail.
That the yielding conquers the resistant
And the soft conquers the hard
Is a fact known by all men,
But utilised by none."*

(An extract taken from the Tao Te Ching)

A good friend of mine from my home island of Dominica, reminded me of the smooth, rounded quality of broken glass when left to withstand the constant motion of sea water over time. In its natural state water heals, refines, and softens the hardest of structures, from rock to sand, and water always finds a way through to reclaim or reach its original source. So, with fibroids these hardened masses emerge from our crystalised thoughts, negative emotions, energy stagnation, suppression, and excess toxins. Therefore, it will take for us to return to that healing state, that moist and cool energy of water, taking time for inner contemplation and mindfulness, in order to work towards eliminating fibroids over time. We will not be able to heal from fibroids without first connecting with that watery energy, which will allow us to become more intuitive, to see where the underlying imbalances and dysfunctions are in our mind, body, and spirit system.

Conventional medicine does not often have this holistic view of healing, and so tends to treat symptoms in an isolated manner. Our body system does not work like that and in TCM, mind, body and spirit are viewed as inter-connected. Many women have turned to TCM as an alternative to conventional medicine, or as a complimentary life aid. Some of the treatments of TCM include: Acupuncture, Massage such as Tui Na, Cupping, Moxabustion, Energy work such as Qi Gong and Tai Qi (Chi) and Herbal remedies.

Uterine fibroids are termed *SHI-JIA* which means stony tumour. The word Shi means stone and the word Jia means mass.

Many women, after years of dissatisfaction with allopathic medicine, have turned to more holistic treatments of fibroids through TCM. TCM studies show that fibroids are caused by excess toxic build-up, genetic organ-deficiencies, diet and excess cold and dampness or excess heat. The research also shows that emotions can play a major role in these excesses and deficiencies.

From a TCM perspective a practitioner would view fibroids in a more holistic way and would apply a range of treatments to shrink and eliminate them. Causes of fibroids would be viewed as follows:

- Mental depression and qi stagnation
- Improper diet and production of turbid phlegm e.g. alcohol, high yeast products etc.
- Attack by, and retention of, pathogenic toxins e.g. cold, dampness, heat, or toxic build-up

All these factors work towards the accumulation of blood stagnation (stasis) and qi stagnation (stasis), and prevent new, rich blood reaching the uterus. This can then lead to significant deficiencies in nutrients reaching the womb area. Qi needs to be regulated and invigorated once it gets stagnated, so that the stagnant blood can be dispersed out through the body. Any energy stagnation can be removed through treatments such as acupuncture or moxabustion (moxa).

The effectiveness of TCM therapies such as acupuncture, energy work and moxabustion to eliminate fibroids, has been demonstrated by clinical trials in China, Japan, the US and in the UK, leading many to avoid invasive surgery. TCM is also used as a complementary treatment alongside conventional treatment, to eliminate pain, inflammation, and other symptoms.

Massage can also be an effective way to release toxins. Using the Lao Gong point which is Pericardium 8 (PC 8), located at the centre of each palm of the hands, to heal, has been quite profound for me as it is known to clear heat and calm the mind and ease the spirit.

Herb treatments have also been noted to be extremely effective in balancing hormones and for fibroid elimination at their early stages when they are quite soft. Here, a good practitioner will use their intuitive relationship with the herbs to decide which herbs would work best for you. They would also take time to listen to your symptoms from an emotional, physiological, and spiritual level, as these are all tell-tale signs which allow them to diagnose and treat. Herbal remedies are potent and effective, as a plant's vital essence or *qi energy* will be the primary agent to allow its chemical properties to affect that of the patient's. As plants are living things, infused with healing energy, they are an essential aspect of nature, as are we. Why then would we not use them to heal ourselves? The Taoist concepts, practices and fundamental way of life was officially repressed, and yet it survives as a life essential for millions around the world, due to its longevity philosophy.

Many of my clients who have incorporated such practices into their day-to-day living, have witnessed the health benefits when working towards fibroid elimination and boosting their general health. To know that we are essentially peaceful in nature, and that we can flow with life challenges no matter what is thrown our way, can create a more yielding, less rigid, and more receptive approach to how we respond, and this brings more harmony to mind, body, and spirit. To learn more about the benefits of Traditional Chinese Medicine (TCM), Taoism, Acupuncture and Acupressure, you can read books, and research online.

Energy Balancing and Its Health Benefits

We cannot dismiss or underestimate the thousands of years over which the science of Qi Gong has been studied by the ancient ones of Kamit (ancient Egypt) and the Naks of Early China. All of life activity is carried out by the life-force energy (qi), and when we align ourselves with this science, we can generate great amounts of energy which can help to heal us and others. This balancing of qi helps to remove stagnation throughout the body and in the mind, and so, is critical for fibroid elimination, and critical that we understand how emotions, bad food etc. can block this energy and lead to masses.

Qi or *Prana* as termed in the Hindu tradition, is invisible, formless, and silent and yet this bio-electrical energy is the very battery of life itself. When the body is filled with this qi energy, we are full of vitality and can achieve a lot. When the body is depleted of this vital energy, we slow down, feel lethargic, blood and energy get stagnated which leads to disease, and things grind to a halt.

Although we come to earth with inherited amounts of this energy when born, we can also top it up through various energy-cultivating exercises, live foods, and correct breathing in clean air. Qi building exercises such as Qi

Gong and Tai Chi are exceptionally good ways of building this energy force and you may want to explore these at a local centre where you live, or you can study them online. When there are imbalances in this qi-energy, then disease ensues.

The words *Qi Gong* mean energy (*life-force*) cultivation of the mind, spirit, and body in a balancing of the Yang and Yin energies within us. This gentle discipline introduces key movements, sounds and colours to balance our energy system in the body. Practitioners understand that when we work within the natural laws, with an understanding that peace, order, harmony, and balance are essential for vital health, we can truly help to heal ourselves and others by bringing the mind and body back to the centre. In this way, we avoid excesses or deficiencies in energy which create blockages in the whole-body system. Please see the appendix for more detailed information about this phenomenal healing exercise. If we do not start from the premise of bringing our body back to peace/homeostasis, fibroids will have a tendency to grow back, and often they can grow back with a greater velocity.

Fibroids are a functional disease, and they take up energy, they feed on toxins that the body cannot dispose of. So, let us start feeding our bodies into wellness and starving the fibroids OUT! The main purpose of non-western medicine is to bring the body back to balance as quickly as possible. Life challenges will happen, but it is important to understand that we can choose how we respond to life situations.

Here are some of the things we can do now:

- Apply moxabustion (heat) to the area between the coccyx bone and anus, to restore proper energy flow. (See a TCM Practitioner)
- Do daily energy work such as Tai Qi (Chi), or Qi Gong exercises such as swimming dragon, to purify, restore the qi, tone the organ systems, and encourage circulation of qi around the body
- Do grounding and polarity work to balance our spiritual and physical state through simply standing on soil, sand, or grass without shoes on. Make sure it is not too cold, as this can create dampness or cold in the body system. Wear shoes if this is the case

We need to get into positive habits such as doing gentle womb exercises daily, such as kegel exercises, to increase our overall qi levels in and around our uterus, and for good hormonal balance and ovarian health. This area can often get stagnated during our menses, or at work; particularly when working with machines such as laptops, mobile phones and fax machines, which send out a great deal of Electro Magnetic Frequencies (EMFs). This can affect your levels of energy, leading to a state of stagnation.

There is an old Taoist saying that states one can live without food for two months, without water for two weeks and only a few minutes without air. Qi Gong, Kundalini yoga and such types of activity will teach you how to cleanse and energise the body's bio-electric fields to bring about detoxification and balance. As a practitioner of Reiki for over 10 years, I have marvelled at the energy intensity level that can be generated by directing qi to areas where there is stagnation, in order to heal Self and others.

Within a TCM framework, and through my own studies and application, I have learnt to have a full appreciation for TCM in shrinking my fibroids, and I also learnt to appreciate how thoughts *(YI)*, lead energy *(Qi)*; and depending on whether we accept negative thoughts or positive ones, will impact greatly on our health and well-being, and on our ability to heal ourselves. So, as part of our healing process, we need to work towards changing the way we think of ourselves, others, and life events, for any treatment to be fully effective. By leveraging the energy obtained through herbs, plant-based foods and therapies, we can get our mind, body and spirit balanced to start healing.

In TCM, fibroids are often termed a *career women's disease,* and I can see that there is some truth in this statement in the sense that many women inform me they do not have much time outside of work for self-care. With all these work pressures, there is one thing we might need to remember, and that is a career does not inherently create stress; we do! A career is not synonymous with stress and disease. It is how we respond to life events which will create the stress response as I explained in earlier chapters. It is us living a life without balance, harmony, and peace and without considering how we eliminate toxins, that can contribute greatly to ill-health. Have we been trained to deal with life from a place of 'threat and tragedy' rather than from a place of peace? What are the activities in our lives which make the body and mind disconnect and feel under-siege?

So, let us start to change our energy, let's start to vibrate on healing frequencies, let's start visualising the things we want to achieve in our lives, and clear away the things that obstruct the way to healing; let's create new opportunities, because what we imagine and dwell on is what we get!

Love and the Energetic Impact of Emotions on Health

Many women I work with also place a great deal of importance on spiritual practices to assist them in health maintenance, and helping them to eliminate negative emotions. Regardless of our faith or religion, or if we have no particular religious beliefs at all, there is ample evidence to show how dwelling on positive, loving thoughts, can change the neuron connections in the brain, and lead to more positive outcomes around our well-being.

Harbouring negative emotions can diminish our life-force energy (qi). You can detect this objectively just by observing your drop in energy when you receive news of a family member passing away, or news about a best friend gossiping about you. The thoughts that we accept can and will determine how we then feel moments later, and it will take some time for the body to return to its original state of homeostasis/balance. Prayer or meditation on loftier thoughts, sentiments and images, can assist us in maintaining this state of inner peace, and this is truly 'medicine' for the body and mind, because it generates the energy required for healing.

Ask yourself what is the key belief you empower each day? It makes sense that emotionality happens most when our consciousness is distorted and imbalanced, and loses its highest vibrational energy, which is LOVE. Are we undertaking loving acts when we act out of anger, jealousy, greed, fear etc? You see, we can do all the right things like eating a vegan diet, doing regular *Qi Gong* or *Tai Chi*, living in a clean environment, using chemical-free products, but if emotions rule our life, then we are still on a pathway to dis-ease!

Many of us are living in societies which often do not celebrate who we are as women, often do not seek to validate and celebrate the feminine, and which constantly super-impose distorted and often unrealistic images of us on the screens. We live in societies which 'rubber-stamp' emotionalism and tells us that anger, fear, grief, jealousy, envy etc. are 'natural' to us; after all, they say, we are only human. We will most definitely need another spiritual and mental framework to stay in the healing zone, amidst what may often appear a 'war zone'.

We are living in environments that encourage excess. We are at crisis levels when it comes to trying to experience balanced vibrational frequencies of peace and harmony, and very often we are not making the correlation between this imbalance, world unrest and internal unrest, leading to dis-ease. Love is truly the universal urge to oneness that every human craves, and it should not be imposed; it is not conditional. In fact, it is an energetic frequency which emanates from us at 528Hz. Yes, we are balls of energy in essence, vibrating at almost the speed of light. When we cultivate gratitude, appreciation, kindness, and humility, we will find that we become loving beings. So, we must change our vibes through meditation, yoga, mindfulness and other practices which seek to bring us back to our true nature.

Hydration - Water, Water Everywhere

One of the fundamental steps we can take as of today, to help towards fibroid elimination is to start drinking sufficient water each day, to assist in our detox process. Yes, it is a solvent, but it has more properties than we realise, and it plays a critical role in maintaining the body's metabolic and water-dependent chemical reactions. Our watery substance in the body creates hydroelectricity which is critical for all of life activity, and life itself; we are electrically charged beings. We fail to realise that when we do not drink enough water (at least 1.5-2 litres of water each day), we are triggering drought in our body system, and dehydration ensues. In much of the traditional healing research cited, deficiency in water is seen to be one of the contributions to social stresses such as fear, anxiety etc. This is because the brain requires water to ensure the electrical energetic communications to various parts of the body flows effectively. Water is a conducting agent for the brain and the cells, and this is vital.

The question we must ask ourselves is, do we see our body as nature's laboratory or the devil's lavatory? Then we can decide to take that step towards detoxing and making the necessary changes in our diet and nutrition for womb-wellness. Everything that creates dis-ease is preventable!

Meditation and Breathwork

The main purpose of holistic health is to bring the body back to homeostasis as soon as possible to aid the healing process; considering the mind, body, and spirit bodies. Meditation has many benefits and one of them is to still and calm the mind, leading to relaxation. However, there is another purpose to meditation and that is to change the way we think, feel and act by reducing the fight-or-flight response to life events.

Breath is life itself and it has many fundamental properties that maintain our health and vitality. It is not just about filling up the lungs with air and then expelling carbon dioxide and other waste products. For many of us, we have not been taught to breathe correctly, and so the shallow breathing has created a great deal of unwellness such as anxiety and hypertension. When delivering lectures around *The Art of Breathing* women often ask me what does breathing have to do with fibroids? It was through my own personal journey of adapting the way I breathe, which brought me to the realisation of just how significant breath is for overall health maintenance, and to aid me in the detoxification process towards shrinking my fibroids.

The first significant thing I learnt is the importance of breathing through the nose and not through the mouth. By inhaling with our mouth, we make ourselves susceptible to viruses, and we are sowing the seeds for the growth of un-wellness. There are no filters in the mouth. The fine hairs in the nostril are a perfect, natural and automatic filtration system; all the debris particles and toxins from the external environment get trapped and prevented from entering the respiratory or blood circulatory system. Part of this breathing process is to not only inhale the air into the lungs, but to take it down into the lower abdomen into the 'sea of breath' which is located 3 inches below the navel, where it is stored.

The blood turns blue and dark as it carries the waste products back to the lungs to get re-filtered by thousands and thousands of tiny capillaries. As we breathe in oxygen, then this oxygen comes into contact with this blood and an amazing combustion process happens where the blood is purified and oxygenated, to then go back to the heart and around the body; purified, rich and full of qi energy. In one day alone a total of 34,000 pints of blood gets oxygenated and purified in this way and so we learn to appreciate the need to stop preventing the body from doing its job. If we breathe through the mouth, this purification and filtration process gets aborted, and under-nourishment and over-toxicity will be the result. Correct breathing has been known to help renew libido, sexual potency, cure ailments, improve mental processes and much more.

If this important life-giving dance to wellness is impeded, we can find that toxins remain in our blood, and the blood becomes dark, stripped of nourishment, and clotty due to stagnation. This type of blood quality is often seen in women who have fibroids. One of the reasons for this is due to the lack of energy and flow of life-force energy (qi) entering the body through our breath.

The body requires about 2,500ml of quality air daily and yet many of us are only taking in 500-600ml. People who do not breathe properly or do not take in sufficient quantities of air will inevitably get unwell. If you notice any changes in your blood quality or menstrual flow, then it is best to share this with your health practitioner as it could be an indication that your blood is not being oxygenated to full capacity, or not pumping through your body efficiently.

It is crucial that we become more familiar with this qi energy term as part of our healing process. In our normal day to day breathing activity, we inhale a certain amount of this energy to keep us alive, however it is only through activities such as lower abdominal breathing, yoga, meditation, and Qi Gong, that we practice breathing which enables us to increase our capacity to take in more qi/energy and to extract and utilise it in greater supply.

Something I have also learnt is that eating on the go or doing other activities whilst we eat, can affect the assimilation of our food. It is advised to take time out to sit and eat and to practice lower stomach breathing whilst eating slowly so that the qi energy from the raw, live, plant-based food, can transfer and nourish our nervous system, digestive tract, and our brain. I mention raw so that it is clear that we can only get large amounts of energy through plant-based foods. More on that in the later chapters, as a balanced, plant-based diet, is a fundamental requirement to assist in fibroid elimination.

Many of us have not even been introduced to this life-sustaining substance called qi, or have dismissed its essential, life-sustaining value. Yet, the first thing some nurses or doctors advise patients to do when they are unwell is to get out of their bed and go for a walk in the fresh air. How does it feel when you walk by the sea with the waves lapping at the shore? Some may say it's exhilarating.

Through the art of meditation, we can learn to breathe deeply through the nose. Watching the level of toxic thoughts that we accept day to day, and the acting out from our thought processes which are either caught up in past or future worries, fears etc, are other ways to help restore our fibroid health. Let us get it straight, thoughts become flesh! They affect our whole physiology, emotions, energy levels, quality of blood, nervous system and hormones; our very cells…yes, our entire body systems. So, let us watch the thoughts we accept about ourselves and each other.

Many of us are breathing incorrectly and this is concerning as we are seeing increased cases of anxiety, hyperventilation, high blood pressure and hypertension amongst women. Incorrect breathing, where we are only activating a small portion of the lungs, can lead to a range of symptoms that we may not initially attribute to shallow breathing, such as frequent sighing, breathlessness, light headiness, a heaviness in the lung area, inability to concentrate, difficulty coordinating our breath, difficulty talking and/or eating, heart palpitations, pins and needles in feet and hands and exhaustion. When we only engage the upper part of our chest in breathing, then we are receiving less or more than the body's requirements. Holistic health practitioners often link incorrect breathing to prolonged stress conditions in people's lives. When we are under pressure for long periods of time this can lead to long-term tension, dilated pupils, sweaty palms, defensiveness, a sense of feeling under attack, increased heart rate, heightened over-reactivity and/or feeling to attack. Yes, breath is key, and a free therapy available to us through the draw of a breath!

Meditation facilitators often guide their patients to start breathing at a slower rate, and to train themselves to breathe through the nose and from the lower abdomen and not the chest, so that they get into a more relaxed state. If the nervous system lacks oxygen, this can create a constant fight-or-flight response and have a negative impact on the nervous system. In previous chapters I mentioned just how damaging this fight-or-flight response can be if too frequently experienced in life situations deemed threatening, worrying, anxiety-ridden, bothersome etc.

Stress lowers levels of melatonin, causing increased growth hormones which stimulate fibroid growth. Stress also raises pro-lactin levels which inhibits the level of progesterone in the body which then can increase levels of oestrogen even further. Hormones are grossly affected by stress levels in our life, and these are so delicately balanced that any change in toxicity can cause major disruptions. So, BREATHE…

In summary, breathing is based on balancing the yin and yang which creates a bridge between the body, mind, and spirit. It extracts qi from the air and drives it through the tiny meridian channels in the body. It is the essential nutrient for the body and is often seen as even more vital than eating or drinking water because it influences the whole body's bio-chemical balancing. When we breathe incorrectly, this impacts the nervous system because the nerves get under-nourished by undernourished blood, lowering the vibrational energy of the nerve currents to the brain, narrowing the blood vessels, leading to less blood flow through the arteries, thereby causing stagnation or clots, dizziness, lack of focus…need I go on?

If our natural balance of breathing cannot be maintained, then the toxins cannot be eliminated out of the body efficiently. Toxins then get stored in fatty tissue cells around the body and can lead to over-toxicity, which can then lead to poor circulation, clots, lethargy, frustration, low libido, irritability, moodiness, cramps, and fibroids.

Cultivating Mindfulness in Meditation

Living in the present is one of the most powerful and life-changing states I have experienced, and I have found that it reduces negative emotions that get trapped in the body through worry, fear, anxiety etc. Cultivating a daily practice to be 'present' in the moment, is truly liberating and prevents thoughts and emotions flooding the system. I recall a previous relationship, where my partner was overly critical of times I chose to go for walks and just watch the water or look at a field of yellow buttercups growing. In Jamaican parlance he would say, "why are you spending time tellin' cow how de do!" It aggravated him as he saw this as time wasting. But it was that need within my inner being to connect with the higher source and just 'be', that seemed to bring me so much intuition, success, energy and so much creativity, and later I learnt it was by living in the present that we tap into, and plug ourselves into, a higher power; the source itself.

Through the cultivation of mindfulness, we can eliminate the ego/mind which constantly strives for power, a winner, and a loser, longing for possessions, to have the last word, pushing for recognition and that special pat on the back, when we can just BE. Just watch the thoughts and choose not to get embroiled and hindered by what they are projecting, do not accept them as you. When we live in the present, we are satisfied, we are complete, we are whole. It is the mind that tells us that we are incomplete, we are not good enough, we are failures, we are unhappy because we do not have this or that, we are denied, we are frustrated, or we are powerless.

In one of my mindfulness classes, early into the session where the attendees expected me to go into a long introduction, I asked the group to just sit and do absolutely nothing for 5 minutes. It was difficult for most of the group to be still. Then, something magical occurred and I observed the changes as the group quietened down. The twitching stopped, the facial tension eased away and there was a release of energy flow around us all. When they opened their eyes and they had an opportunity to share, many mentioned that it was a powerful experience to connect back to themselves. During the activity, they became more aware of their surroundings; the room, the energies in the room, the sound of the clock ticking, the bird singing outside the window; they became aware of how tense they were and could identify where this tension resided. They all promised themselves to practice the exercise daily as part of their regime in the morning and to offer gratitude in their renewed self-awareness of the power of being present. It truly was magical! Try it!

Yes, we know EVENTS happen! But the key thing to acknowledge is that we can respond differently to life situations and change our mind-set about whether we see the event as against us, a threat, or as an opportunity for us to grow. Our thoughts and ideas, when repeated enough times, become belief systems and these can become crystalised. They can become the framework or premise by which we live our lives. Think about it; do you feel the world is a safe place or a threatening place? Do you dwell on a lack of safety and lack of protection daily? Do you feel you deserve to be loved and to be accepted? In other words, what are the internal scripts you hold on to and how are they playing out in your life?

All physical events in our world are directly controlled by the life-force energy (qi), which in turn, is controlled by what resides in our minds. Consequently, our self-image and what we project daily is critical, as it determines what we create through our projections. Yes, fibroids are created!

Here is a simple breathing exercise I personally find extremely useful. Breath therapy is known to help assimilate and circulate vital energy, extract toxins from tissues, stimulate hormone secretion, purify the blood, and massage your organs and glands. So, here goes...Breathe!

1. Sit in an upright chair with your back straight
2. Create a slight curve in your back
3. Breathe in through nostrils for a count of 4, slowly and steadily pushing your lower abdomen out (1, 2, 3, 4)

4. Hold for 4 (1, 2, 3, 4)
5. Breathe out for 8 (1, 2, 3, 4, 5, 6, 7 ,8), pulling your lower abdomen in

Repeat this for 5 minutes

The Deep Sleep

When supporting women who have fibroids, I spend quite a bit of time introducing them to the circadian cycle. This is a cyclical rhythm of our internal body clock, which controls our body's functions throughout the day and night. It has been interesting to note that the vast majority are not aware of this cycle, and if they are aware of it, have not been trying to structure their life around the cycle for optimal health. For example, the liver detoxification process starts at between 1-3am in the morning, and many women are still awake or working shifts, which greatly impairs the liver organ system to do its job of detoxification. There is a 'master clock' situated in the hypothalamus which synchronises neural and hormonal signals such as hormone release throughout the day.

It is important to recognise that we can often hinder these natural processes and stop them from working optimally. Another important reason for reducing or cutting out caffeine or coffee, is that it blocks the adenosine receptors which affect sleep and wakefulness. When we sleep, adenosine levels rise up again ready for the waking state in the morning, and the melatonin levels go up to prepare you for the stages of the sleep cycle. This cycle is divided into 90-minutes of rapid eye movement (REM) and non-rapid eye movement (NREM), which gets repeated throughout the night. During the NREM stage N3, the deepest sleep stage, the body does its growth and repair activities. This stage assists the body to restore energy to the brain and body. It is critical that we do not sabotage Mother Nature's gift of reparation through our sensual and material urges to go out drinking, partying, watching late night movies, etc. It is advised that women aged 26-64 years old get between 7-9 hours of sleep (National Sleep Foundation).

Inadequate sleep has been associated with a variety of health problems; in the short-term these include fatigue, impaired learning and memory, and irritability. Adequate sleep is necessary for a healthy immune function. Consistently depriving yourself of sleep can lower your immune system and make you susceptible to illnesses such as the cold and the flu.

40% of women have a higher risk of insomnia than men, and if not addressed it can lead to mental, emotional, and physiological health problems such as mental fatigue, muscle fatigue, impaired learning and cognition, hypertension, and irritability. Sleep controls our stress hormones and maintains the nervous system. Many women I have spoken to over the years have not made the connection between sleep and their general health. Very few had regular 8 hours of uninterrupted sleep due to work patterns, insomnia, family life, young children, watching TV late at night or other lifestyle choices.

It is important to recognise that in wanting to eliminate fibroids, we need to regulate our sleep patterns and understand that a lack of sleep can lead to imbalanced hormones. Progesterone levels can drop when women have fibroids, and they can also drop if women are experiencing stress responses to life challenges. If progesterone drops then oestrogen can rise, and may lead to what is termed 'oestrogen dominance'. If the correct ratio and fine balance between these two hormones is not achieved, then this could lead to an inability to fall asleep, or to have uninterrupted sleep. Progesterone is a sleep inducer, as well as assisting your breathing during the sleep process. If it starts to drop, then women can often feel very fatigued throughout the day, leading to relationships and productivity suffering, and a feeling of not having rested at all the following morning.

You may benefit from seeing an endocrinologist for a test. The concerning risk is that people who sleep less than 5-6 hours per night, are twice as likely to develop diabetes. Speak to your GP about testing your progesterone and oestrogen levels, because properly-balanced progesterone in women will alleviate emotional imbalances such as mood swings and fogginess, as well as encouraging a stronger immune system, better conversion of stored fat into energy, and peaceful sleep. It will also yield healthy oestrogen levels, which are key to reducing the likelihood of fibroid formation and growth.

These are things that we women need to consider in order to get on track with our sleep; adhering to the circadian cycle without disruption or with minimal disruption; trying to remain consistent with the amount of sleep Monday to Sunday, so that we don't break the cycle at weekends with a lie in; turning the mobile phone onto aeroplane mode or off at night before bed; changing the screen colour on our phones to reduce melatonin suppressing light; stop watching TV by about 9pm; avoiding late night snacking and eating; avoiding coffee or stop drinking it after 1.00pm; and trying not to work on laptops and desktops after 7.00pm.

A Relationship with Self - Tuning in and Body Awareness

A fundamental part of eliminating fibroids is having a positive relationship with ourselves. We can grow in our understanding of how interconnected we are to everyone and everything around us and start creating healthier friendships.

I am BEING – composed as a duality. We must understand SELF/Energy/Matter, to function well in the world. The most important thing in the healing process is to be true to your own essential nature, and that is peace!

Make time for contemplation and get to know our minds and bodies. Release! If there are any changes, get checked out. Some of the early signs of fibroids may be numbing pain, heavy, increased, or prolonged periods (menses). We want to catch fibroid development early, to have a better chance at elimination and to avoid invasive surgery.

"A peaceful woman,
Does not seek anything,
Does not push for anything,
Does not try to please anyone,
Does not compete for anything,
Does not yearn for anything,
She just IS…and all that is for her comes effortlessly"

By Imani Sorhaindo (Auraum Benneurt)

Feminine Sexual Energy

As women, it would be beneficial to learn just how fundamental our sexual energy and vitality are, as part of staying vital, healthy, and creative in life. Creative and Spiritual energy are one and the same, and many different communities and religious institutions shy away from speaking about sex and sexual energy in a healthy way. This can often suppress and oppress women by making them think it is separate and sinful. Womb-wellness is all about creating balance in this area of our life. How do you feel about your sexual energy? When you feel that surge of energy rise up in you, what do you do? What have you been taught about sex and sexual energy? The energy can be cultivated and then directed to different parts of your body, to aid in healing, so one must question why societies would want to deny anyone their expression of sexual energy. More and more women have asked me about a range of treatments which are known to assist in improving sexual energy, libido and womb-wellness, as well as general vital health. These include Yoni pearls, Yoni steaming, Womb Cleansing, Castor Oil packs, Eco-Pads and Yoni eggs, to name a few. I have not undertaken sufficient research for this book to comment on many of these, although I have found yoni steaming and castor oil packs have been beneficial for my own reproductive healthcare.

Sisters! health, and vitality are the source of good sexual energy. It is no surprise that many women who have fibroids start to feel lethargic, turned off by sex or plain tired. Blood, energy, and vital nutrients are leaked out of the body during each and every menses, and we need to replenish these and let go of the toxins. When we hold things in or suppress feelings such as, hurt, rejection, neglect, frustration, feeling unappreciated and unloved, feeling a lack of nurturing, then we can experience health problems within the uterus area. It is truly time to heal!

Inducing Joy

Yes, there is a great need to tap into our pleasure principle, to enjoy our life experience. Most women I speak to each week are not enjoying life and we often search for happiness outside of ourselves. When this happens, if we lose the thing we thought we needed for happiness, we sink into depression and frustration until the next 'thing' that seems to bring us happiness comes along. This mode of thinking is creating a great deal of anxiety and depression in the lives of many.

There is a principle within every one of us that allows us to connect with a state of joy at any given time, purely through the images we accept and hold on to each day. It is an aspect of us that allows us to enjoy things, harmonise with others, flex a little with life, and be more sociable. Are you connecting with this? It is in us already! It is not outside of us. So, the questions we must ask ourselves are, how joyful are we each day? What is our capacity right now to be joyful? What are we waiting for to feel joy?

An example of this is our approach to waking up each morning. Do we jump out of bed dancing with abundant gratitude and joy for being here another day or do we always flood our mind with negative images and words about what we think the day ahead is sure to bring us? This is all within our control, based on the choices we make and our thoughts. Is it going to be Joy or Pain? When we start to recognise that an event is neither inherently stressful nor pleasurable, but it is just an 'event', we begin to get a glimpse of our liberation. Whenever we see something as 'terrible', 'awful' or 'stressful', instead of seeing it as an opportunity, then we have already handcuffed ourselves to images of gloom and despair. This triggers the production of toxic chemicals in our body system, which can then trigger off oestrogen excess, if continually occurring.

So, in a meditative state, we can cultivate this joy faculty to visualise images which evoke pleasurable sensations. This in turn, floods our body with the most healing, happy hormones, to create a state of calm and relaxation. Let us make a choice today, positive vibes or negative vibes? Let us not starve the joy. In one of my classes on *The Art of Mindfulness*, I worked with a woman who was constantly experiencing panic attacks when going into work to complete tasks. She started each morning with images of failure and feelings of dread. These images and words prevented her for months, from enjoying her breakfast with family and her walk to work. She could not even remember what colour the flowers were on her way to work or who she saw. By the time she got to work, her mind and body had already shut down and she was tense and apprehensive.

Through creative visualisation we worked together to create pleasurable images of her day, which slowly reduced her negative symptoms. The results were positive as she started to relate to herself, her family and work colleagues differently, which then changed the negative outcomes she was preparing for each day. In the sessions she learnt that joy is an energy state, and we are in control of arousing it through a range of activities and sensations (sounds, images, scents, words). It works on a vibrational level, which in turn affects the brain waves and chemical reactions in the brain. Slowly she started to work with essential oils, colours, and meditation CDs in her home, to keep the powerful work going. Therefore, we must feed the joy to heal and stay healed.

CHAPTER 8
Diet, Nutrition and Supplementation

It is no wonder our health is in a mess when we think about what enters our digestive palate and gut every day. Some of the foods which are known to be antagonistic to maintaining a healthy internal system are very often the foods many women struggle to cut out. Some holistic health practitioners refer to these foods as 'alarm' foods. If you come away from reading this book and decide to make just two changes in life, then let them be correct breathing and diet! I cannot urge women enough to consider seriously that certain alarm foods are literally sending the body into a state of arrest daily, due to their unnatural properties which conflict with nutrition, digestion, and absorption. These include white sugar, white flour, white pasta, white rice, artificial sweeteners, GMO products, processed foods, alcohol, meat, and refined oils like sunflower and canola etc. Yes, these are all 'dead' food!

We Become What We Eat

What we eat, how and where we eat, can be key determinants to our health and longevity. There is a science to eating which many of us are not taught, and this can create havoc in our minds and in our bodies. 'Live' food is a consideration as part of fibroid elimination. The truth is, if you want energy, go to the source which takes in over 90% of that life-force energy (qi), from the sun; plants!

In books written about ancient history and spirituality, there are frequent references to herbs, healing foods, or foods for the wise. Spirituality, live food, and wellness, go hand in hand, and yet many of us will ignore the call from nature to come back to the centre. Good health can also start in the gut, as it is deemed the second brain. Eating quality food, and being able to assimilate and digest this food, are all key parts to staying healthy. Bacteria, mould, and fungi build up and dwell in this wonderful environment and co-exist harmoniously until we get in the way of this balance. Imbalances can create headaches, depression, skin problems, allergic reactions and more. We may also need to consider pro-biotics to assist in maintaining good gut health.

We are electric people, yet most of what we eat can diminish our electrical, energetic capacity and it is no wonder we feel lethargic and imbalanced. Minerals also determine the quality of life that we live and yet how many of us are actively seeking to bring balance to our lives with minerals? A live body needs live foods, rich in minerals and vitamins, and yet we are eating so many foods which create starch, mucous and excess toxins.

The minerals in the earth are depleted due to high levels of chemicals, and this should be concerning us greatly. The body will only heal itself and fully maintain healing itself, when the food we eat reflects nature.

There are many schools of thought that show disease begins in the colon and in the gut, and is caused by mucous. Gut health is critical for any revolutionary change in terms of reducing fibroids, and in general wellness for all, therefore it is best to decide to start growing and/or buying food which promotes good gut health and aids in the digestion and assimilation of food. Fermented foods are great for gut health, as they regulate the gut flora by introducing good bacteria into our system. Food such as non-GMO fermented tofu, kombucha, kimchi, are just a few to get started with as an introduction. Green tea is also a great way to initiate the detoxification process in a nice, gentle way. It can be drunk 1hr before meals to get the body ready for digestion and assimilation.

Many of us, myself included, did not take much notice of the colon as part of any health strategy initially, yet toxic build up in the colon is life-threatening because the colon can get blocked with mucous instead of being fed by oxygen and water that it needs to stay healthy. The 'alarm' foods are oftentimes, blocking the way.

Mindful Eating

Mindfulness eating can be practiced to maintain and develop clear-thinking, assimilation of food and assimilation of ideas, good digestion, and toxic elimination. To accompany this practice, we can work with Qi Gong or yogic exercises which strengthen the spleen and stomach organ system.

One of the things we can get better at, is slowing down our eating, to chew many times to better absorb the food, aid digestion, trigger the secretions which help to break down the food and aid in the elimination of toxicity. The mouth is the first organ to receive our food and if we are eating live food, then we are absorbing the etheric particles of the food, as well as the denser particles of food. We start to appreciate that we need to have more of a spiritual connection with the food we eat, to absorb the life-force energy (qi). Some considerations:

- Always try and eat in silence as much as possible; however, I appreciate that family mealtimes also bring pleasurable and healing sensations to the mind and body
- Stop talking and eating at the same time
- Stop multi-tasking when eating
- Hold warm and pleasurable thoughts as you visualise the food nourishing you
- Eat 'live' (plant-based) foods as much as possible
- Do not use food as a punishment or comfort and do not eat when angry

Eating in this way will help you connect to the live food you eat, and to nature. It will start to generate feelings of appreciation and gratitude within you. We must remind ourselves that fibroids are the body's way of saying we are not connected with ourselves and to nature, and there is some foreign agent, whether it is our thoughts, emotions, a chemical or hormonal substance, pervading our body system, which is creating excess oestrogen or toxins. Eating is one of the ways that we can remain connected to nature and our natural vibrations.

I have fond memories of my childhood in Dominica, including mealtimes and get-togethers with family and friends when we gathered to eat and share. This sharing of such warming energies around food is beneficial and they continue to evoke strong memories, which even now, stimulate the 'pleasure hormones' and aid healing. Yet, many of us may not have this type of relationship with food. Food may have been used as a punishment in childhood, or a day-to-day hustle or challenge because of finances. We may just shovel it in without much thought or care, or are not cognisant of its life-giving properties as we go about our day. So, it may take a revolutionary act to change the 'dance' we have with food.

Ok, now let me introduce you to live foods or power foods. All food has what is termed an *energetic temperament*. Foods are governed by planetary energies and have a special therapeutic function. Live foods are vegetables, nuts, fruit, seeds and grains, which contain high levels of living enzymes. Live food such as fruit and vegetables are rich in a condensed form of solar energy. This is great, but our body has to be receptive and in a vital state to be able to absorb all this energy and utilise it to aid healing. This can be a mindfulness meditation that you take time to do when you eat, which you will find powerful and energising. As we start to take time to contemplate on the purpose of life, we start to make different choices about what to think and act upon, what to eat, what lifestyle to have. Would you rather eat at a restaurant where the staff have created the food with the sole intention of making a profit by any means necessary or would you choose a restaurant where the staff spend their time and energy ensuring the food leaves you feeling even more vitalised and nourished?

Enzymes have life-force energy (qi), and are required for digestion and assimilation. Fried foods or foods which have been cooked at extremely high temperatures, destroy these enzymes, and end up pulling on the bodies reserve supply, leading to daily ageing. This aging occurs when we do not replenish the body with these enzymes and life-enhancing properties, leading to symptoms such as lack of energy, lack of memory, greying of hair, loss of libido and weak bones. A pear or an apple is 100% live food when freshly picked. They contain 80% water and foods with higher water content are termed *alkaline foods* which are also particularly good for us. When we then cook, bake, or stew these foods, they lose much of this energy, despite the apple crumble having more appeal than just eating a raw apple.

It is also important to maintain a spiritual connection with the food that we eat, and this is difficult if eating processed food. There are foods which we will get to learn about that feed and nourish the 7 parts of our make-up (Cosmic, Nirvanic, Etheric, Spiritual, Psychical, Astral, and Mental). Such live foods act as healing agents and have the highest amount of qi energy. When we are unwell, these foods will be able to affect the mind, body, and spirit positively, whereas allopathic drugs can only affect us on the physical level. It is important to recognise that to eliminate fibroids we need to change what we eat and how we eat, to manage and restore our health. I would suggest that there are 10 key things around food to consider and act on if we really want to heal ourselves.

These are:

- Recognise that we are what we eat,
- Try out new plant-based recipe options and make it fun, not a chore,
- Start a gentle detox of the body (one day a week to start with),

- Introduce organic foods into your diet,
- Eliminate GMO products,
- Eat clean proteins, not mock or processed foods,
- Introduce green juicing daily,
- Introduce supplementation. (There are 3 types of supplements we need to factor into our daily regime: multi-vitamins, multi-minerals, and antioxidants),
- Have peace in your mind when preparing, cooking, and eating your food,
- Explore alternative medical treatments (Chinese herbs, homeopathy, acupuncture for example) to work in a complementary way alongside your healing foods.

Nutritional Therapy

Nutritional therapy is critical towards the elimination of fibroids. Who would think that a simple fruit such as a pear is so invaluable in the healing process? The pear is renowned for its excellent properties in preventing and reducing fibroid tumours and other benign growths. This is due to its high content of a phytonutrient called *ellagic acid*, a mineral called *boron*, and an insoluble fibre called *lignin*. These compounds work synergistically to aid our healing, bringing the body back to wellness. I encourage you to explore fruit and vegetables which reflect the colours of the rainbow. After a recent lecture I attended on the *Cosmogony of Health* by Dr Tau Napata in London, I was motivated to seek out the nutritional content of each of these rainbow colour foods. Below is a list I researched but it is not exclusive:

Purple: prunes, plums, grapes, cherries, cabbage, blueberries

Red: watermelon, tomatoes, apples, beets, cranberries

Orange: carrots, pumpkin, mango, cantaloupe, apricots, sweet potato, peaches, satsumas, papaya

Yellow: lemons, pineapple

Green: limes, peas, peppers, cucumbers, kiwi, avocados, lettuce, beans, kale, cabbage, Brussels sprouts

So, let us have some fun with food! Gift yourself a green juice smoothie!

Ingredients:

- ½ cantaloupe melon
- Small piece of ginger (* Optional as some clients with lupus or other health conditions are not advised to have ginger)
- 1 apple (organic)
- Handful of washed organic kale
- Handful of washed organic spinach
- Bottled spring or filtered water or freshly squeezed orange juice (0.5litres)
- ¼ lemon
- Little pinch of cayenne pepper
- 1 stick of celery
- Sprig of parsley

Indole 3-Carinole

This is a phytonutrient found in most cruciferous vegetables such as broccoli, kelp, Brussels sprouts, purple or white cabbage, savoy cabbage, red bell peppers, Chinese cabbage, onions, and ginger. Kelp is also great for dissolving fibroid masses and reducing blood and energy stagnation. These foods are great antioxidants and anti-tumour agents as they are good at blocking the negative effects of excess oestrogen by promoting oestrogen to beneficial metabolite levels. This phytonutrient is known to lower the risk of breast cancer and the production of fibroid masses. Indole 3-Carinole stimulates the phase 2 enzyme system that helps to clear cancer-causing toxins from our body, it is seen as protective to oestrogen-sensitive tissues and may be beneficial to people with health issues related to oestrogen dominance.

Sulforaphane

This component in certain foods such as broccoli, broccoli sprouts, Brussels sprouts, and cauliflower, triggers natural cancer-blocking agents in the body. It helps rid the body of harmful stress and alarm signal molecules. In relation to broccoli sprouts, it is interesting to know that 3-day old sprouts contain 20-50x more of this chemical than the matured sprouts, and if you steam or boil them this chemical is greatly reduced. The best way to utilise it is to grate the above vegetables finely and mix into your salads or lightly steam.

Essential Fatty Acids (EFAs)

Something that you need to consider is starting to eat foods which are high in EFAs such as sea greens like Nori, which is high in iodine and rich in B12. Other foods include spinach, cantaloupe, avocado, and olive oil. Brown algae, seaweed and kelp are all softening agents and many women have been known to shrink fibroid masses by consistently having these EFAs in their diet. Evening primrose oil is also a good form of EFA. Sea vegetables are high in chlorophyll, which is a substance in plants that have certain health benefits as we align closer to nature when we eat them. These EFAs help to renew tissues, invigorate and re-build blood, improve liver health, detoxify the body, remove any drug deposits from our system and reduce and relieve inflammation. Most wholefood stores will have a range of these green foods such as: blue-green algae, chlorella, alfalfa, wheat grass and barley. Examples of sea vegetables include agar, arame, dulse, hijiki, kelp, nori, and wakame seaweed. Evening Primrose oil or borage oil are also great ways of ensuring you have enough EFAs in your diet.

Gluten-Free Foods

Yes, this was one my challenges! For many of us brought up on bread as a staple diet, it is something we have to consider adjusting in our diet if we want to shrink fibroids, as wheat has been noted to set off an allergic reaction because the gluten is indigestible for many people. Although you may not be experiencing severe symptoms, you may still have a gluten insensitivity or intolerance. Check it out with your GP. There are mild symptoms which may include dizziness, pain, bloating, flatulence, and depression.

For many, food has become nothing more than an inconvenience. Where some strive to educate themselves about food to have a healthier lifestyle, for others food simply 'gets in the way' of our day-to-day productivity and our financial and work goals. Food is so often seen as something we shovel in and excrete out, plain and simple, and yet, we fail to understand, and are often not given the information to gain an understanding, that it is quality food which powers our physical, ethereal, and psychical bodies. It is the yin part of us which nurtures and powers the external yang side of us, consequently our relationship with what we eat, and importantly, how we eat, is pertinent here. Eating has become such an unconscious activity that we are not truly maximising the healing process of eating and aiding the digestive process to fully benefit from the properties of food. As I write this, I start to visualise my kitchen being transformed into a food magnificent healing haven.

Supplementation

One of the areas which we need to act on is the level of supplementation we take in daily, due to the poor quality of the soil which grows much of our food, depending on where we live. This is due to environmental factors and chemicals in the soil. Speak to your GP about the foundational supplements to take for optimal health.

Some of the key supplements for women's health include:

Vitamins A, B12, B complex, C, E, D3, B6: help the liver to metabolise oestrogen properly, and minerals such as magnesium, selenium, iron, zinc, calcium, magnesium (night-time). B12 is also required for gut health and for good thyroid health which can really assist in hormone balancing.

Vitamin D is critical for fibroid elimination as this hormone is known to have anti-tumour properties. You can get Vitamin D tests done, so explore this with your GP.

Magnesium and zinc get depleted when food is processed, and they are responsible for over 500 essential body functions.

Antioxidants such as Dehydroepiandrosterone (DHAE), which also balances out your mood, folic acid, alpha lipoic acid (a great liver detoxifier), N-acetyl cysteine (a powerful detoxifier), Omega 3 oils (pour on rice or salads) and iodine.

Fenugreek supports HGH and testosterone yang build up to improve libido.

Pau' d' arco is also a powerful anti-tumour herb which helps to breakdown fibroid masses. Turmeric has anti-inflammatory properties. Ginseng can be used for stamina and vigour. Astragalus can be used for spleen and for gut issues or for loose stools if your spleen /stomach is compromised.

Glutathione plays a vital role in liver health and aids the detoxification process. It is excellent for boosting your immune system. Take with alpha-lipoic acid. Alpha lipoic acid helps the body to regenerate. It is a great free-radical scavenger!

C0-Enzyme Q10 which is an energy-producing substance.

If drinking coffee at all, it is advised that you have this at least 6 hours before bedtime as this can affect the level and quality of sleep. We need deep REM sleep to take us into delta or theta state of sleep to aid healing. Some attending my coaching sessions have found that having their last meal at least 2 hours before sleep has also been impactful. Food can interfere with the release of growth hormones which we need daily to keep us youthful.

Tinctures such as black cohosh is an oestrogen balancer for fibroid relief. Dandelion herbs help to stimulate the liver, to metabolise excess oestrogen, reduce breast swelling and stomach congestion. Dong Qua and Tang Kwe are master Chinese herbs to nourish women during their menses and enrich the blood and qi energy.

The benefit of fasting is so vast I cannot cover it fully in this book, however I encourage everyone to spend a day a week at the very least fasting on live, green organic foods, lots of orange juice and water and a good liver cleanse. There are also cycles such as the Equinox and Solstice periods in the year when it would be beneficial to fast for longer periods, and practitioners in the back of the book can guide you.

Remember to check with your GP or a qualified health practitioner before following any of the recommendations in this book. I would always encourage a thorough holistic healthy diagnostic assessment as it is not a one-size-fits-all approach recommended for healing the mind, body, and spirit.

CHAPTER 9
Concluding Remarks - A Wake-Up Call for Health and Wellness

There is a law that states that for every action there is an equal and opposite reaction. We now need to search for and choose the right actions, to yield the lifestyle experiences we truly yearn for. Yes, we can remain at the hands of our GPs and medical institutions only, and they do a good job in the main, however, true and full healing comes from within and it's in our hands.

Looking at all the research gathered, and working with so many women experiencing fibroids, I would strongly recommend that a higher focus and intervention needs to be placed on preventative information and better-informed self-management strategies, in addition to the existing crisis–management which appears prevalent. Bearing in mind the 2012-2013 statistic of 30,000 hysterectomies carried out in the UK that year, the situation is rising and often times not being reported because of reasons I have already highlighted in previous chapters. How are we educating ourselves and the next generation to make more informed choices?

If you are a woman with fibroids, but not experiencing major symptoms at this early stage, it would be best not to just sit back and watch them grow. The softer and earlier stage in formation, the easier they are to be eliminated, so act now! Fibroids, big or small, are a sign that the body is out of balance and needs detoxification. Doctors may suggest you do nothing and wait and watch; monitoring them with scans along the way, however 80% of women I interviewed said they wished they had taken early action, and wished they knew about some of the non-invasive strategies much earlier on. 100% of these women experienced their fibroids growing much larger within 3-12 years after their early detection.

Earlier in the book I made the correlation between womb-wellness and productivity because more and more women are having to balance full-time motherhood with full-time employment, and this often means neglecting their health. Recent research shows that women spend between 6-10% of the time off work dealing with the symptoms of their menses alone. This is increased further by 15% when issues around fibroids and endometriosis come into the picture. We need to start seeing this as an issue that not only affects women, but the whole planet, and it is through sharing the information about holistic approaches to healing that we may find answers.

Another useful step is to keep a journal and note down incidents which create tension in your life, foods which aggravate, mind or body changes, so that you become far more self-aware. This will help you be more informed when speaking to your GP, and for them to be able to share all the options available to you. It is important for you to be an active participant in your well-being, and not a passive bystander. Do your own research about the range of treatments out there, and the dietary, mental, and emotional factors which cause fibroids to grow and accelerate in growth.

There are lifestyle changes you can start to take now, which will be life-changing for you and those around you. Do not let the only time we focus on health be the time when we have lost it! Start to place YOU top of your agenda, and the world will treat you differently. Remember that the more invasive treatments come with the highest risks, so think seriously and carefully through your options.

Getting Started – A Checklist for Fibroid Elimination

*Note: With any change to your diet, consult your healthcare practitioner. Keep a journal and jot down your reflections. Share any changes or improvements in your energetic, mental, and physical system with your physician. A holistic practitioner would take all these aspects into consideration when guiding you towards health improvements.

General Fibroid Healthcare

- Seek guidance around how to make castor oil packs to reduce or eliminate fibroids,
- Consult a good homeopath, herbalist and acupuncturist as these treatments work well together,
- Consult your health practitioner about enzyme therapy, such as introducing protease, which helps to dissolve and reduce abnormal tissues, and helps boost the immune system,
- Avoid or reduce the number of x-rays you have, such as mammograms

etc. Ask for an ultrasound scan first if there is a need for a check,
- Consider a T4 test to check the blood level of the hormone T4 (thyroxine) as this may be an indication of hormonal imbalance,
- Avoid contraceptive pills as they are high in oestrogen.

Self-Care

- Create space for YOU in your busy life,
- Learn to meditate or pray,
- Drink more water (2 litres a day),
- Sleep 8 hours a night. Not in the day. Follow the natural cycles of life, be in tune with nature's plan,
- Obtain regular full body massages to help eliminate toxins from the lymph system,
- For painful menses, take tissue salts such as Kali Mur and Kali Sulph,
- Keep your weight in check. There are links between obesity and fibroid growth and accumulation,
- Research the best essential oils which are made from pure extracts from plants. There are some products which have phenomenal properties to aid healing fibroids as well as for general health and well-being,
- Create rest time between the times of productivity,
- Avoid getting addicted to work,
- Cultivate daily gratitude about the good things in your life to feed those happy hormones,
- Watch your words and thoughts, and try to identify and eliminate the root causes of triggering emotions which become real-life monsters in your life (I am agitated, I am irritated, I cannot help losing it, I am a mess, I am niggled, I am out of sorts, I am frustrated, I cannot take it etc.)
- Get to know your body. If there are any changes, get checked out. Some of the early signs may be numbing pain, heavy, increased, or prolonged periods (menses). You want to catch fibroid development early,
- Look at the ingredients in creams, hair, beauty, and body products. Start to choose a chemical-free and organic product range.

Exercise

- Avoid high impact exercises such as jumping for long periods as this can put a strain on the joints, ligaments, and tendons over time. Consider activities such as walking, bouncing on a trampoline, light running, cycling, swimming and rope jumping. Exercise is a stress reliever and

helps balance the hormones and gets rid of excess oestrogen and progesterone,
- Start breathing correctly. We need to take in at least 2,500 ml of oxygen daily. Practice deep lower diaphragmatic breathing,
- Exercise for at least 30 minutes daily. Sweat!

Nutrition, Diet and Supplementation

- Avoid white bread and limit wheat bread as they produce mucous. White bread has a lot of chemicals and sugar and can create insulin spikes in the body,
- Try and alternate between sprouted breads, pumpernickel, or rye or better yet, bake your own bread and research the quality of the flour to avoid aluminium-soaked flours due to processing,
- Eliminate or greatly reduce alcohol intake which disrupts hormones,
- Eliminate meat, particularly non-organic meats, which create fatty tumours and cysts. There are growing concerns that red meat doubles the risk of developing fibroids. Pork also has the highest number of parasites which can destroy the healthy micro-biome in the gut,
- Eliminate hydrogenated or refined oils which often go through a great deal of processing to become solid or spreadable, and do not fry foods in these oils, as they are highly carcinogenic,
- Follow a low glycaemic index (GI) diet plan,
- Limit or eradicate processed food such as white pasta and other floury products - all are heavily refined,
- Eat organic fruit and vegetables, especially dark green organic vegetables rich in chlorophyll. Wash any non-organic vegetables in a non-chemical-based veggie wash or apple cider vinegar and not under tap water which often has a lot of heavy metals,
- Eliminate dairy products such as dairy cheese, milk, and ice-cream,
- Mushrooms promote uterine health,
- Eat more cruciferous vegetables (broccoli, cauliflower, cabbage, Brussels sprouts),
- Avoid cold drinks which can damage the spleen/stomach function,
- Make green juices with spinach, kale, chlorella, or spirulina and add chicory, apple, and ginger,
- Drink cleansing teas such as red clover, burdock, golden seal, dandelion and green tea. Many of these have anti-inflammatory properties that help to metabolise excess oestrogen,
- Daikon radish is renowned for its properties which help to move qi

energy around the body,
- Don Qui is great for women under 50. It helps as a blood builder after the loss of key nutrients through menses. It builds up the iron and helps with anaemia, which is one of the symptoms often caused by fibroids,
- Peony is also good for anaemia,
- Eat foods which are high in EFAs (Essential Fatty Acids) such as sea greens like nori, which is high in iodine and rich in B12. Other foods include spinach, cantaloupe, avocado and olive oil. Brown algae, seaweed and kelp are all softening agents. Borage and Evening primrose oil is also a good EFA,
- Black cohosh is also great for balancing hormones naturally,
- Holy basil has been used by some clients as an adaptogen which helps to reduce stress hormones built up in the body. Ashwagandha also lowers cortisol hormones in the body,
- Bacopa Monnieri which is an adaptogen, supports mental alertness and hormonal balance,
- Alternate between almond milk, oat milk and soya-based products, which seem to have higher oestrogen levels,
- Reduce caffeine, chocolate, and sugars, which tend to aggravate fibroids and aid toxic build up,
- Read up more on alkaline foods, as opposed to highly acidic foods and make the necessary changes.

Vitamins and Supplements

- Get your Vitamin D3 – Sunshine or through supplementation
- Take your daily supplements. Vitamin C, B12, B6, B Complex, D3 and K2, Zinc and Iron.

∞ APPENDIX 1
Useful Resources

Holistic Centres

Khamitic Therapeutics Ltd
Integrative Holistic Health Centre – This Centre has a large product range in women's essence, restoration, sexual vitality, fertility, supporting endocrine health and reproductive health. They also have their own bespoke herbal tinctures that cover a wide range of women's health issues, together with supportive health, spiritual wellness and mental health counselling.
Email: info@khamitic-therapeutics.com

Introducing the Khamitic Therapeutics Team
Mr Tau Napata – CEO & Director of Services
Spiritual Counsellor, Naturopath, Homeopath & Alternative Therapies Practitioner; Qi Gong Master – Specialising in Energy Cultivation Practices through his dynamic programme *NuShuRa*

Clinical & Therapeutic Services Team
Head of Clinical Services - Ms. Muku Qesua Wilson - Integrative Holistic Practitioner
Specialising in Homeopathy, Herbology, Nutrition and African-centred Psychotherapy as well as Women's health, Endocrine imbalances & Restorative work.

Ms. Khesu Abba Saa Seshem - Integrative Holistic Practitioner
Specializing in African-centred Birth Partnering Services and Support, Herbology, Female Energy Cultivation & Restoration Practices, Spiritual counselling with a particular focus on Family Services and Support.

Holistic Practioners

Tarze Edwards-Small - QiLife- A Holistic Health Company
TuiNa Medical Massage speeds up the body's ability to heal itself, moving

stagnation and increasing mobility, relieving joint pain, muscle spasms, by stimulating oxygenated blood flow. TuiNa Medical Massage Complements Qigong.

Qi Gong - Healing Qigong, is preventive and self-healing. As such it can help rejuvenate organ energy systems like the endocrine system which becomes overtaxed by menopause, dysmenorrhea, vulvodynia and other female health conditions.
Email: support@qilife.co.uk
Website: www.qilife.co.uk
Instagram: @Senbisa

Olivia Haltman (OHServices)
Integrative Counsellor and EMDR Therapist
Services provided (internationally online):
- Counselling
- Emotional Impact of Fibroids Sessions
- EMDR
- Workshops
All services are holistic and used with an integrative approach as we believe everyone has different needs, therefore we create the service to the clients' needs.
Email: ohservices@counsellor.com
Website: www.ohcounsellingservices.com

Dr Patricia Smith (Kamit Health)
Services offered: Physiotherapy, Massage, Acupuncture and Chinese Herbal Medicine.
Email: kamithealth2021@gmail.com
Website: kamithhealth.com

Valerie Mcken – Womb Wellness Warrior
Email: Valeriemcken@gmail.com

KMT Rising Ltd Holistic Health
Imani Sorhaindo - Holistic Health Practitioner, offering person-centred coaching for fibroids. On-line service and women's support groups in London
Email: kmtrisingltd@gmail.com
Website: www.kmtrising.com

Other Well-being Consultants

Noire Wellness
The Noire Wellness Fibroid Series is a 12 week health education programme to help women reduce the effects and manage the impact of fibroids. A blended delivery of online and face to face offer is available depending on location.
Email: info@noirewellness.com
FaceBook, Twitter & Instagram: @NoireWellness
Website: www.noirewellness.com

Useful Websites

www.globalfibroidalliance - Be part of our campaigns and awareness raising world-wide. Get in touch at GFA2020@mail.com
www.info@thelakefoundation.org
www.thewhitedressproject
www.nhs.uk/conditions/hysterectomy/pages
www.healthline.com
www.hormonesbalance.com

Twitter Sites

@drSydneyjd
Dr Syndney Dillard, Ph.D.; Associate professor at DePaul University has dedicated her life to addressing fibroids.

@lakehealthwell
A non-profit organisation that aims to improve the health and well-being of local, regional and online communities.

@OH Services
Counsellor and Course facilitator supporting women around the emotional impact of fibroids.

@fibroidforum
A very useful site that raises awareness, shares information and supports women with fibroids.

APPENDIX 2
Bibliography

Articles

Ashpari, Zohra Ashpari and Cirino, Erica. Medically reviewed by Natalie Butler, RD, LD, May 2017

Burden, Prevalence, and Treatment of Uterine Fibroids: A Survey of U.S. Women

Bosland, Maarten C. et al. Effect of Soy Protein Isolate Supplementation on Biochemical Recurrence of Prostate Cancer After Radical Prostatectomy: A Randomized Trial. The Journal of the American Medical Association, Vol. 310, Issue 2, pp. 170-178, 10 July 2013

Carrafiello G, et al. Cardiovasc Intervent Radiol. 2010. PMID: 19777299

Dallas, M.E. Hysterectomy May Have Long-term Risks. Health Day News. Wednesday, Jan 3, 2018

Haney AF. Clinical decision-making regarding leiomyomata: What we need in the next millennium. Environmental Health Perspectives. 2000; 108 (Suppl 5): 835-839. (PubMed).

Hezel, Francis X. The cult of the individual, SJ, Micronesian Counselor, Edition 65, January 2007

Hiroshi, Ishikawa, et al. High aromatase expression in uterine leiomyoma tissues of African-American women, J Clin Endocrinol Metab, The Endocrine Society, 95(5):1752-1756, Feb 2009

Journal of Women's Health, Volume 27, No.11, 2nd November, 2018

Kjerulff KH, Langenberg P, Seidman JD, Stolley PD, Guzinski GM. Uterine leiomyomas – racial differences in severity, symptoms, and age at diagnosis.

Journal of Reproductive Medicine. 1996; 41 (7): 483-490. (PubMed).

Lee, Sang-Ah. et al. Adolescent and Adult Soy Intake and Breast Cancer Risk: Results from the Shanghai Women's Health Study. The American Journal of Clinical Nutrition, Vol 89, Issue 6, pp. 1920-1926, June 2009

Levy. Barbra S. Acta Obstet Gynecol Scand. 2008

Martin-Merino, et al. The reporting and diagnosis of Uterine fibroids in the UK: An Observational Study. BMC Women's Health, 2016

Messina, Mark. Soybean isoflavone exposure does not have feminizing effects on men: a critical examination of the clinical evidence. Fertility and Sterility, Vol. 93, Issue 7, pp. 2095-2104, 1 May 2010

Morito, Keiko. et al. Interaction of Phytoestrogens with Estrogen Receptors Alpha and Beta. Biological and Pharmaceutical Bulletin, Vol. 24, Issue 4, pp. 351-356, April 2001

Parker, WH. Etiology, symptomatology, and diagnosis of uterine myomas. Fertil Steril 87:725-736, 2007

Tucker, Katherine L. et al. Simulation with Soy Replacement Showed That Increased Soy Intake Could Contribute to Improved Nutrient Intake Profiles in the U.S. Population. The Journal of Nutrition, doi: 10.3945/jn.110.123901; 27 October 2010

Ultrasound-guided radiofrequency thermal ablation of uterine fibroids: medium-term follow-up,

Wilson, Wendy L. ESSENCE MAGAZINE 2009 Health and Fibroids

Wu, A H. et al. Epidemiology of Soy Exposures and Breast Cancer Risk. British Journal of Cancer, Vol 98, Issue 1, pp. 9-14, 15 January 2008

Books

Amen, Ra Un Nefer. Qi Gong Healing Prescriptions, Khamit Media Trans Visions, New York, (2009)

Amen, Ra Un Nefer. Qi Gong Success, Khamit Media Trans Vision, Inc, New York, USA, (2009)

Amen, Ra Un Nefer. Tree of life Qi Gong: Volume 1: Balancing Heaven and Earth, Khamit Media Trans Visions, New York, (2004)

Appleton, Nancy. Lick the sugar habit, Avery Penguin Putman, New York, (1996)

Baker, Sidney Macdonald. Detoxification & Healing: The key to optimal health, Keats, New York, (1997)

Batmanghelidj, Dr. F. Your Body's Many Cries for Water: A revolutionary Natural Way to Prevent Illness and restore Good Health, Tagman Press, London, UK, (2000)

Black, Jessica. K. (ND). The Anti-Inflammation Diet and Recipe Book, Hunter House Publishers, Canada, (2006)

Campbell, T. Collin (PHD) and Campbell, Thomas. M II. The China Study, Benbella Books, Texas, USA, (2006)

Chia, Mantak. Healing love through the Tao: Cultivating Female Sexual energy. Huntingdon, Healing Tao Books, New York, (1986)

Chia, Mantak. Taoist ways to transform stress into vitality, Healing Tao Books Inc, New York, (1996)

Brannen, Barbara Ann. Hands of Light: A guide to healing through the human energy field, Bantam Books, USA, (1987)

Daniel, P. Harnessing the power of the universe Reid, Simon and Schuster, London, (1998)

Dossey, Larry. Healing Words, Harper Collins, New York, (1993)

Dreher, Diane. Women's Tao Wisdom: Ten Ways to Personal Power and Peace, Thorsons, London, UK, (1998)

Duffy, William. The Sugar Blues, Chilton Book Company, (1975)

George, Mike. The Immune System of the Soul: The Journey from Awareness to Realization to Transformation and Freedom from A Dis-ease, Gavisus Media, Dubai, (2013)

Goodwin, Scott C., (MD). What your doctor may not tell you about fibroids, Warner books, New York, (2003)

Jackson-Dean, Dr. L. M. (DM, MBA). Seeds to Change – Systematic Oppression and PTSD, (2017)

Lao Tse. Tao Te Ching, (Translated by Arthur Waley), Wordsworth Editions Ltd, (1996)

Levy, Thomas. E. (MD., JD). Curing the Incurable, Livon Books USA, (2002)

Liu, Da. The Tao of health and longevity, Routledge, and Kegan Paul, London, UK, (1978)

Northrup, C. (Dr). Women's bodies, Women's Wisdom: The complete guide to Women's Health and Well-Being, Piatkus Books, UK, (2020)

Omraam Mikhael Aivanhov. The yoga of nutrition, Collective Izvor, Prosveta Editions. (1986 2nd Edition)

Perkins, Cynthia (M ED). Break your sugar addiction today, Cynthia Perkins Publications, USA, (2013)

Pert, Candace, P. Molecules of Emotion: Why you feel the way you feel, Simon & Schuster, 1999

Segal, Inna. The secret language of your body: The secret guide to healing, Blue Angel Gallery, Australia, (2010)

Strom, Max. A Life worth Breathing, Sky Horse Publishing Inc, New York, (2010)
Thompson R, MD and Barnes, K. The Calcium Lie Vol II: What your doctor still doesn't know, Take Charge Books, North Carolina, (2013)

Van, Andre, Pranayama: The yoga of breathing, Lysebern, Unwin Paperworks, London, (1971)

Watson, George (MD), Bantam Books, New York, (1972)

Young, Dr Robert O. (PHD) and Redford Young, Shelley. The pH Miracle: Balance Your Diet, Reclaim Your Health, Wellness Central, USA, (2010)

Zakhah, Israel. The Joy of Living Live: A Raw food journey, Communicators Press, (2005)

∞
INDEX

Acidic foods 16-17, 84
Adaptogenic herbs 14
Adrenals 11-14, 20, 29, 30, 34
Alkaline 16, 18, 74, 84
Anaemia 4, 5, 84
Aromatase 33, 34, 88
Ausarian vi
Balance/d xiii, x, 1, 4, 12-19, 25-30, 39, 41, 45, 49, 51, 52, 54, 56-59, 62-64, 67, 68, 71, 72, 78,-80, 82-85, 87, 92
Black women iv, xi, xii, 7, 8, 33-37, 39, 40, 42, 44-46
Bleeding viii, 3, 4, 7, 14, 48, 50
Breath/ing iii, x, 14, 17, 26, 29, 40, 56, 60-67, 71, 83, 91
Calcium 5, 17, 22, 23, 32, 78, 91
Causes iv, x, 1, 16, 19, 24, 34, 55, 82
Cervical fibroids 3
Circadian cycle 66, 67
Coffee 11, 16, 23, 66, 67, 79
Contraceptive pills 25, 51, 82
Cryomyolysis 50
Detection 4, 6, 42-44, 80
Dis-ease x, xii, xiii, 7, 9, 11, 17, 20, 21, 25, 31, 41, 47, 48, 53, 56-60, 72
Dopamine 10, 19
Drugs 1, 12, 19, 20, 25, 31, 40, 43, 50, 74, 77
Electro Magnetic Frequencies (EMFs) 24, 26, 58
Environmental toxins 7, 9, 13-15, 22, 24-27, 29
Essential Fatty Acids (EFAs) 77, 84
Exercise xii, xiii, 15, 20, 56, 57, 65, 72, 82, 83
Fatigue 25, 38, 39, 48, 66, 67
Formaldehyde 25, 41
Genetically Modified Organisms (GMO) foods 20, 21, 23, 24, 71, 72, 75, 83
Gluten 77
Hair Relaxers 40, 41
Harmony vi, 15, 28, 52, 56-59
Herbs 5, 14, 25, 43, 54, 55, 58, 71, 75, 78, 79, 81, 85, 86
Holistic v, vi, ix-xiii, 1, 8, 27, 33, 45, 51, 52, 54, 55, 60, 63, 71, 79, 81, 85, 86

Hormones 10-15, 20-22, 29, 30, 40, 48, 55, 63, 65-67, 70, 73, 78, 79, 82-84, 87
Hyaline Degeneration 5
Hysterectomy viii, ix, xi, 6, 7, 42, 44-49, 80, 87, 88
Imbalances x, xii, 1, 4, 12, 14, 16-18, 25, 27, 28, 39, 41, 45, 54, 57, 59, 60, 67, 71, 72, 82, 85
Indole 3-Carinole 76
Inflammation 10, 15, 17, 19, 49, 50, 55, 77, 90
Intramural fibroids 2
Joy 18, 27, 32, 34, 37, 69, 70, 92
Kidney 3, 15, 16
Liver 9-12, 15, 17, 21, 27, 30, 31, 66, 77-79
Meditation 14, 28, 59, 60, 62-64, 70, 74
Menses/Menstruation viii, 4, 5, 12, 43, 45, 58, 68, 69, 79, 80, 82, 84
Mindfulness 28, 54, 60, 64, 65, 70, 72, 74
Moxabustion 54, 55, 57
Myomectomy ix, 7, 44, 48, 49
Natural vi, ix, 5, 9, 10, 14, 15, 19-22, 26, 27, 30, 34, 40, 45, 52, 54, 57, 59, 61, 64, 66, 71, 73, 76, 82, 84, 90
Neurotransmitters 19, 25
Nutrition xii, xiii, 10, 13, 14, 17, 20, 60, 63, 71, 75, 83, 85, 89, 91
Obesity 15, 20, 21, 47, 82
Oestrogen 1, 10-15, 21, 24, 30, 31, 33, 34, 41, 48, 50, 51, 63, 67, 70, 73, 76, 78, 79, 82-84, 89
Parabens 26, 40
Peace vi, vii, x, xiii, 1, 13, 27, 28, 30, 39, 52, 53, 56-59, 67, 68, 75, 90
pH 16-18, 26, 92
Plant-based food 14, 22, 58, 62, 73, 74
Pollutants 9, 25
Post Traumatic Slave Syndrome (PTSS) 34, 38
Post Traumatic Stress Disorder (PTSD) 34, 91
Progesterone 12-15, 48, 63, 67, 83
Racism 27, 34-39
Risk 4, 7, 9, 15, 16, 22, 25, 47, 48, 50, 67, 76, 81, 83, 88, 89
Sex 4, 12, 43, 45, 61, 68, 69, 85, 90
Sexual Energy 68, 69, 85, 90
Sizes viii, 1, 2, 4, 6, 23, 33, 43, 44, 47, 51
Sleep 12, 19, 66, 67, 79, 82
Spiritual iv, vii, 31, 36, 51, 52, 55, 57, 59, 68, 71, 73, 74, 85
Submucosal fibroids *fibroid diagram*, 2
Subserosal fibroids *fibroid diagram*, 2

Sulforaphane 76
Sulphates 40
Supplementation/Supplements 5, 7, 25, 46, 71, 75, 78, 83, 84
Symptoms viii, x, 4-8, 12, 14, 19, 25, 34, 39, 42, 43, 45, 47, 49, 50, 53-55, 63, 70, 74, 77, 80, 84, 88
Traditional Chinese Medicine (TCM) 1, 27, 53-58
Thyroid 14, 30, 48, 78
Toxic Overload 10-12, 17, 18, 21
Toxins xi, 1, 7, 9-11, 13-15, 17, 18, 22, 24-27, 30, 31, 39, 51, 54, 55, 57, 58, 61, 64, 65, 69, 72, 73, 76, 82
Trauma 31, 32, 34, 37,38
Treatments ix, x, 1, 2, 4, 5, 7, 8, 33, 34, 43-47, 49, 50, 51, 54, 55, 58, 69, 75, 81, 88
Types *fibroid diagram*, 2-4
Uterine Artery Embolization 49
Vibrational 13, 28, 50, 52, 53, 59, 64, 70
Water xiii, 9, 17, 19, 25, 26, 37, 52, 54, 58, 60, 64, 72, 74, 76, 79, 82, 83, 90
Womb-Wellness vii, viii, xiii, 14, 60, 68, 69, 80

NOTES

Printed in Great Britain
by Amazon